Miguel Angel Troiano
Mauricio Benincasa
Patricia Sanchez

Dental Implants.Inmediate Loading Full Arch. New concepts

AF209875

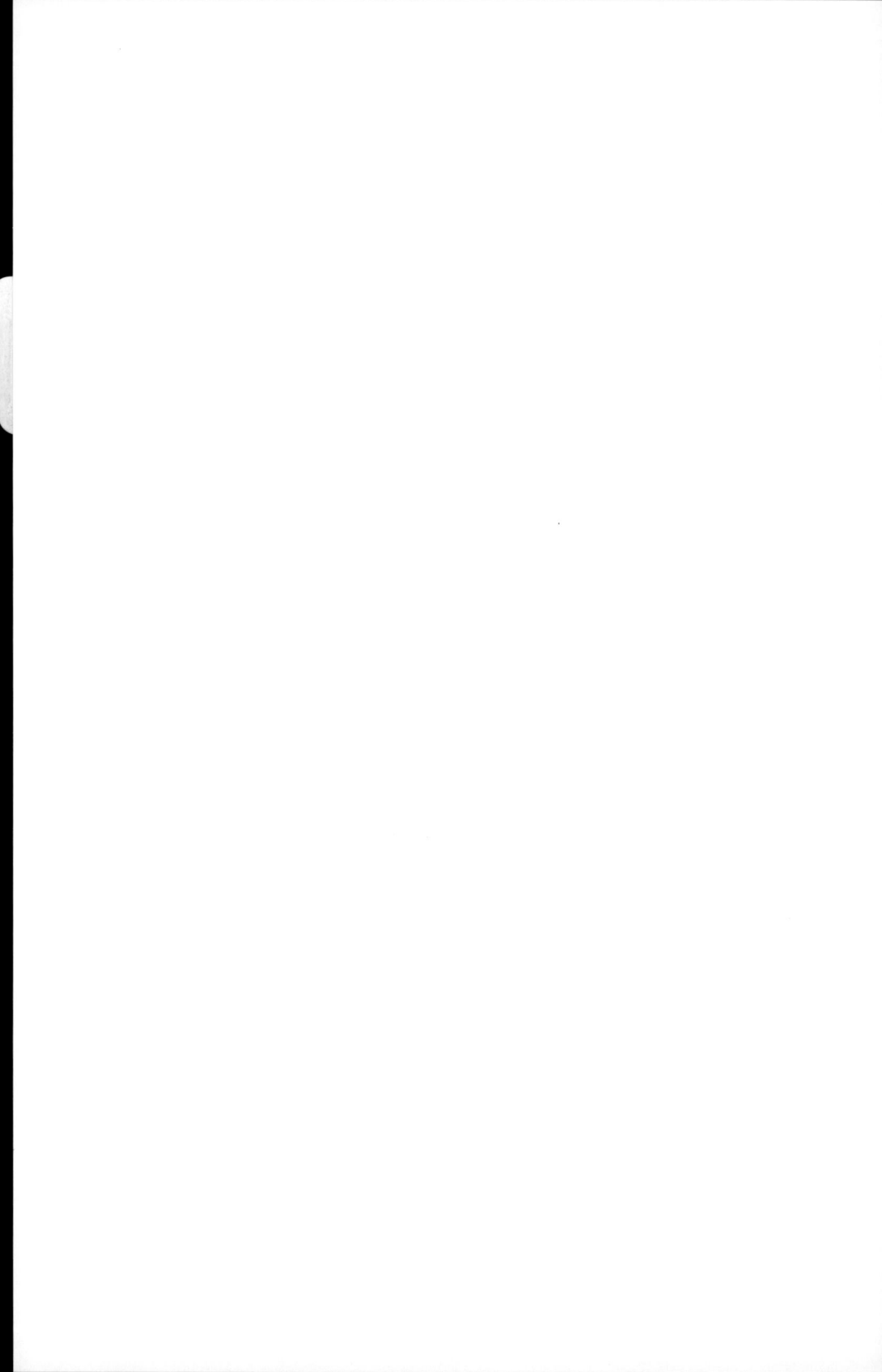

Miguel Angel Troiano
Mauricio Benincasa
Patricia Sanchez

Dental Implants.Inmediate Loading Full Arch. New concepts

LAP LAMBERT Academic Publishing

Publisher:
LAP LAMBERT Academic Publishing
is a trademark of
Dodo Books Indian Ocean Ltd. and OmniScriptum S.R.L publishing group

120 High Road, East Finchley, London, N2 9ED, United Kingdom
Str. Armeneasca 28/1, office 1, Chisinau MD-2012, Republic of Moldova, Europe
Managing Directors: Ieva Konstantinova, Victoria Ursu
info@omniscriptum.com

Printed at: see last page
ISBN: 978-3-659-11443-4

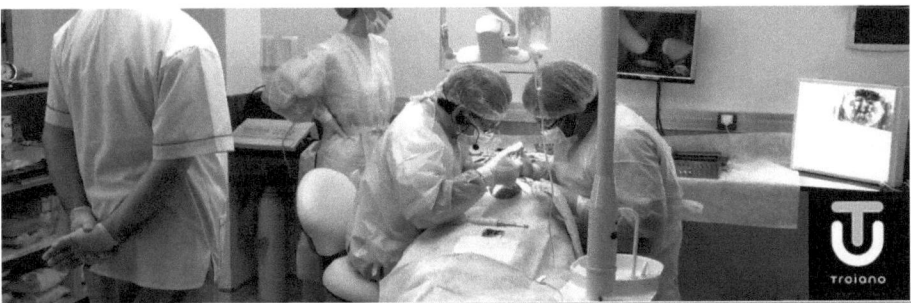

DENTAL IMPLANTS. INMEDIATE LOADING FULL ARCH. NEW CONCEPTS

Miguel Troiano

Patricia Sánchez

Mauricio Benincasa

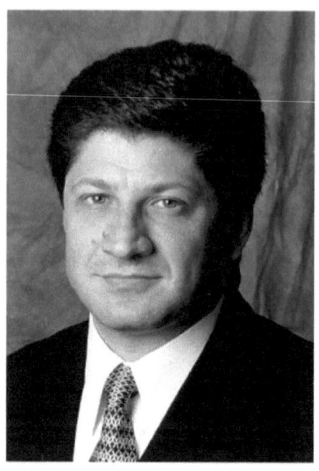

Author: Miguel Angel Troiano

- Graduated from the Faculty of Dentistry of Rosario.

- Teacher Specialization in Prosthetics and Rehabilitation dentobucomaxilar Integral Implantoasistida. (University of Buenos Aires).

- Lecturer at courses, conferences and clinical charts in Argentina and abroad

- Member of the American Academy of Osseointegration

- Member of the European Academy of Osseointegration

- Member of the American Academy of Osseointegration

- Member Partner Specialist Argentina Prosthodontic Association. Sectional Argentina Dental Association

- Author and co -author of several scientific publications in Argentina and abroad (Brazil, Uruguay and Europe)

- Co- author of "Oral Implantology Actual Approach"

- Co -author and editor of the book "Immediate Loading on Prostheses Implantoasistida. Biological Bases and Therapeutic Applications"

- Member of the International Committee of the Journal editor Dental Dialogue

- Member of the International Committee of the Journal editor Annals of Oral & Maxillofacial Surgery

- Affiliate Member by invitation - Publication Ethics & Integrity (P.I.E.)

1

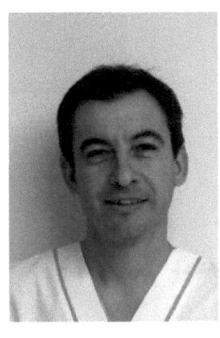

Co–author: Benincasa Mauricio

Graduated from the Faculty of Dentistry of Rosario.

Specialist in High Complexity Prosthetics Rehabilitation with Orientation in Implant -assisted prosthesis and Fixed and Partial Prosthodontics.

Member of Argentina Prosthodontic Association.

Sectional Argentina Dental Association.

Author and co-author of several scientific publications in Argentina and abroad (Brazil and Uruguay)

Co–author r of the book "Immediate Loading on Prostheses Biological Bases and Therapeutic Applications"

Member of Troiano Odontología Institute.

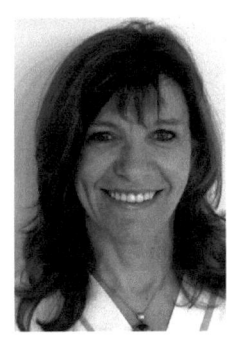

Co–author: Sánchez Patricia

Graduated from the Faculty of Dentistry of Rosario.

Member of Argentina Prosthodontic Association.

Sectional Argentina Dental Association.

Specialist on Endodontic.

Author and co-author of several scientific publications in Argentina and abroad (Brazil and Uruguay)

Co–author r of the book "Immediate Loading on Prostheses Biological Bases and Therapeutic Applications"

Co–director of Troiano Odontología Institute.

Dental Implants. Inmediate Loading Full Arch. New concepts

Generality

For the last two decades, dental implants have been regarded as a predictable means of achieving oral rehabilitation. In retrospect, this seems to be due to three main factors: the biocompatibility of titanium, the design and surface of the implants and the receptivity of the host. Since the 1990s, two other elements have been added to the list and have been changing constantly: surgical technique and load conditions.

The original two-stage Branemark protocol developed in the early 1970s (Branemark et al 1977; Branemark et al 1985) has been gradually modified, leading to the one-stage surgical protocol (Berlungdth et al 1991-1994, Abrahmson (1996-1999), which has become standard procedure. This was made possible by the detailed study of bone-healing stages carried out by Schenk et al (1990) that proves that an implant loaded occlusally over a 6 month period is loaded into bone tissue which has already healed but is still immature, given that bone maturation takes 24 months.

With this in mind, industrial biotechnologists have modified the surface of the implants, thus accelerating osseointegration, which now takes from 45 to 60 days and is referred to as "early loading."

Consequently, osseointegration can now be passive or active.

Furthermore, implant macro- and microgeometry has become extremely important for a successful treatment (Szmukler-Moncler et al 1996). The surface of the implant must be structurally similar to the surface of the bone, which has evolved over 450 million years (John Davies 2006).

Osseointegration, discovered and tested by Branemark in the 1970s on animals and later on humans in the 1980s, is a biological reaction to a surgical action. This triggers a series of systematic and automatic restorative response mechanisms: the first protein to enter into play is thrombin, which enables the formation of a clot; the second one is fibrin, with which the repair process begins.

When the surface of the implant is flat, it retracts, leaving a space between the surface and the bone tissue, which must be filled with Osteoblast to achieve osseointegration in 3 to 6 months. This is known as "passive osseointegration," discovered by Branemark in the 1970s. In the 1990s, a number of leading companies developed prepared surfaces, which were divided into two types:

1- With lining

2- Without lining

1- *With lining:*

Applying different elements to the surface of the implant:

a) Titanium-plasma coated (TIP)

b) Hydroxylapatite-coated (HA)

The result was a 20-micron pore that accelerated osseointegration but was detrimental in terms of implant exposure, since the presence of bacteria would lead to peri-implantitis, which was hard to heal. As a consequence, the implants would have to be removed, given that the area could never be properly cleaned due to the size of the bacteria--1 or 2 microns.

Hydroxylapatite is different in that osseointegration is achieved through calcium bonds between the lining biomaterial and the patient's bone, when placing the hydroxylapatite on the titanium surface. This phenomenon was called "biointegration," which at the time of its discovery was considered to be faster and more efficientbut was later seen as problematic because, after a while, the hydroxylapatite would fall off of the surface of the implant and become a bone sequestrum between contact surfaces.

2- *Without lining:*

Essentially, it consists of applying a subtractive technique on the titanium surface, so that porosity will increase and improve osseointegration.

- A. With surface sandblasting (RVM) (blasting the surface with sand, salt, or any other coarse or fine particle)
- B. With acid etching on the surface (osseotite) (simple or double acid etching)
- C. With sandblasting plus acid etching
- D. With titanium particles

These new surfaces meant a modification in the integration mechanism due to a surgical action, which the body identified as an aggression. The ensuing process was the following: thrombin created a clot, fibrin adhered steadfastedly to the surface of the implant, thus creating a pathway through which the osteoblast reached and adhered itself to the surface more rapidly, accelerating osseointegration, which was now possible at 45 to 60 days. This was known as active osseointegration---Buser et al (199 1), Klokkevod et al (1997); Cochran et al (1998); Davies et al (1998); Baker et al (1999); Lazzara et al (1999); Trisi et al (1999); Cordioli et al (2000); Testori et al (2002).

Presently, sector companies are searching for ways in which to improve osseointegration.

The first new approach is nanotechnology: the surface of the implant must be similar to that of the bone, the structure of which has evolved over 450 million years.

After placing the implant, the bone tissue migrates from the medullar area to the implant surface, where microtexture and lamellas help it to creep onto it. Modifying implant topography enhances this effect by keeping microporosity at one micron and achieving a nanometrical separation between particles, the gap being so small that it becomes difficult to tell apart the surface of the bone from that of the implant when looking at a microphoto taken with an electrical microscope which enlarges the image 50.1 to 70.000 times. In effect, the first breakthrough in this field is nanotopography, i.e. the structural topography of the surface.

The second innovation is the technique of surface impregnation of calcium phosphate at a molecular level, which creates an exchange of calcium ions between bone and implant. This method is currently under analysis; experimental studies have already been carried out on animals and shown a 160% increase in osteoconduction, which implies greater bone apposition, greater anchoring and more tensile strength.

Randomized and prospective multicenter studies of the different techniques (immediate loading, one-stage and two-stage surgical approach, etc.), focusing on different parts of the jaw, have already been carried out on humans and the first results are to be published shortly.

At present, the connection between bone and implant is a physical one, but a chemical bond is being attempted, generated by the contact between the platelets and the calcium phosphate surface. (John Davies, Journal Biomaterials 2005)

This is aimed at achieving a type of biointegration which will generate a new bonding system as a result of the exchange of calcium ions between the surface of the implant and the bone.

The technique of immediate loading of implants in full mandibular arches was the first therapeutic attempt at reaching this goal with a high predictability rate.

One of the first to implement the technique were Schnitman et al (1990), who developed a protocol that was named after them.

The team carried out preliminary research and treated two patients, who were examined in one of the centers included in the study. The patients received both implant types--submerged and immediate-load--according to the 1990 protocol, which was adopted in order to ensure placement of a sufficient number of implants in case all immediate-load implants should fail.

This study constitutes a milestone in the field of implantology and was taken up by many other authors: Berlungdth et al (1995); Balshi & Wolfinger (1997); Schnitman et al (1997); Tarnow et al (1997); Wohrle et al (1998); Branemark et al (1999); Ericsson et al (2000); Jaffin et al (2000); Lozada et al (2000);Testori et al (1999); Darvanapah et al (2000). All of the latter agree that, for immediate loading, it is best to place the implants in the supracrestal area.

Testori et al (2001a; 2002b) published two case reports involving both submerged and immediately loaded implants, the screws of which had been inserted into the bone crest, i.e. in what is know as a "crestal position." In both cases, the temporary prostheses supported by immediate-load implants were placed four hours after surgery. After two months, a prosthetic surgery was performed (please see articles for further information) to remove two submerged implants and an immediate-load implant from one of the patients and, four months after the initial procedure, two immediate-load implants were removed from the other patient, which were subjected to a histological examination. All the immediate-load implants showed evidence of bone-implant contact; this suggested that immediate loading does not prevent osseointegration. Furthermore, crest bone loss was similar for immediate-load and submerged implants at every assessment stage.

New prosthetic components have simplified the process of devising restorative structures, making it possible to solve clinical problems more rapidly and efficiently. With an ever-growing range of designs that favor internal connection, clinical practice is facilitated by avoiding inconveniences such as the loosening or breaking of screws.

Machined components for external or internal connections are now more accurate, their rotation and dislocation resistance being greater than ever. Moreover, modern adjustment screws facilitate an appropriate preloading.

Therefore, prosthetic restoration is more predictable and less prone to loosening, while also lowering the risk of structural micromotion--which can affect osseointegration-- giving greater stiffness to the entire structure.

The main goal of an immediate load protocol is, thus, to decrease the number of surgical procedures and shorten the time between surgery and prosthesis placement without affecting implant success rates.

As a result, general practitioners are forced to innovate and modify surgical techniques to improve and accelerate restoration, which benefits the patients and themselves. To achieve this, it is extremely important to devise the best possible treatment for each case in order to obtain the most accurate prosthetic solution in the shortest period of time.

If a new clinical procedure is duly documented and supported by a wide number of cases involving extensive follow-ups and high success and viability rates within normal parameters ensuring predictability, the procedure will eventually become a standard practice.

As regards immediate loading, it can be defined as follows: According to Dr Dennis Tarnow, it is an implant that is subjected to functional occlusal forces from the very first day of placement. This is a basic definition which served to create the technique of immediate loading of implants in full mandibular arches (1994).

For the load to be regarded as immediate, the occlusal implant must be functional within a period of 0 to 7 days. This technique has become routine.

Two landmark conferences were held on the subject: the 2002 Barcelona Consensus, which characterized an immediate load as one carried out on the same day of implant placement (Aparicio et al 2003), and the 2003 Gstaad Consensus, which set the maximum loading time at 48 hours after implant placement (Cochran et al 2004).

Based on the aforementioned parameters, the difference between immediate load and other techniques may be said to be the following:

- **A.** If the prosthetic restoration remains infraocclusal or does not achieve contact, it is not considered immediate loading. If the implant is placed in a one-stage surgery in which an abutment and a temporary crown are inserted, it is viewed as an immediate prosthesis or an immediate temporization procedure.

- **B**. If the prosthesis is inserted 3 weeks after implant placement, it is called primary early loading.
- **C**. If the implants are activated prosthetically at 45 to 60 days, it is called secondary early loading.

In order to observe the osseointegration principles suggested by Branemark in 1985, it is necessary to bear in mind:

- 1. The biocompatibility of the material, in this case titanium –whether or not it is a harmless material that does not affect the immune system
- 2. The design of the implant
- 3. The surface
- 4. The particularities of each case, i.e. the state of the bone
- 5. The availability of a perfected surgical technique
- 6. No loading during the healing process

Immediate loading breaks away from traditional implantology.

The most obvious difference relates to biomechanics, since osseointegration is achieved before prosthetic restoration and thus the biological aspect is given precedence over mechanical considerations. As stated by Dr Meltzer, this technique is actually mechanical-biological. Elements are fixed by means of mechanical devices (implants-components-screws) in order to achieve biological success (osseointegration).

Following this literature, we suggest a protocol that contains seven critical aspects, which serve as a parameter to measure the success and probability rate of a rehabilitation procedure.

1. ACCURATE DIAGNOSIS AND TREATMENT PLAN

In some cases, it is necessary to do a diagnostic wax-up and to establish viable surgical guides to assess the prosthetic area and make all necessary considerations regarding the vertical dimension, esthetics, phonation, smile line and gesticulation– essential aspects when devising a temporary prosthesis.

Radiology (panoramic and periapical x-rays, CTs, 3D-imaging) are also important to ensure a more precise prosthetic surgery, since they allow dental professionals to establish the most appropriate location for the implant, thus making it easier to devise a final immediate prosthesis for each patient after having achieved osseointegration.

2. IMPLANT LENGTH

Implant length must be at least 10 mm and ideally 13 to 15 mm, given that the success of the procedure is closely linked to primary stabilization during placement.

3. BONE QUALITY AND QUANTITY

Type II bone is ideal for clinical applications, since it has very good irrigation and a low risk of bed overheating.

Type III bone is no longer contraindicated in view of the implant surface treatments available today, but in this case the implant must be at least 13 mm long.

Patients with Type I bone are not a serious problem, but good irrigation–if possible, internal and external--is essential for carrying out an osteotomy of the bed; to that effect, disposable, high-speed steel burs should be used: since they are sharper, lower prep time and make for a less invasive procedure, given that they enable professionals to restrain implant length to 10 or 11.5 mm, thus preventing bone overheating. In these cases, a greater number of implants should be used to cover the anteroposterior area and optimize the prosthetic design by achieving a more efficient distribution of occlusal forces in the prosthetic structure, therefore avoiding the use of cantilevers and eliminating parafunctions, or keeping them to a minimum.

4. IMPLANT INSERTION

The advisable implant insertion range is from 30 to 40 Ncm. This is the ideal torque, which generates the right amount of friction, helping to avoid bone overheating and guaranteeing primary stability.

Implant arrangement, parallel placement, bicortical support, separation rate, direction and abutment are extremely important, as is the type of immediate prosthetic connection used.

5. TEMPORIZATION

The temporary prosthesis must be structurally stiff. This enables a better distribution of occlusal loads and a more efficient absorption of forces; additionally, it keeps implants from breaking during osseointegration, which could hinder the process, or altogether prevent it.

There are two types:

- Screw-retained
- Cement-retained

A. Screw-Retained Prosthesis:

This technique is ideal, since it ensures prosthesis retention; it is unlikely for the prosthesis to budge after immediate temporary load placement.

All temporary components must be adjusted by means of screws, with a mechanical or digital torque wrench, applying a torque of 20 Ncm or more for screws with a hexagonal head and a torque of 32 Ncm for those with a square head. Thus, they are virtually impossible to loosen up.

B. Cement-Retained Prosthesis:

This prosthetic structure must be reinforced by an internal or lingual metallic structure to prevent them from breaking, given that the cement is applied on temporary abutment posts placed over the implants, which are in turn screwed in as previously mentioned. The prosthesis can only be removed for implant monitoring after two months.

6. PROSTHETIC DESIGN

The implants must be placed in the two quadrants of the inferior maxillary bone, considering these are full arches that extend over the midline, which is why the resulting forces push towards the tongue. The opposing structures used in prosthetic restoration help to control the forces exerted on vestibular-lingual, mesial-distal and occlusal-gingival surfaces.

Having sufficient anteroposterior space for implant arrangement is essential for implant predictability, as is bearing in mind the antagonist arch and the parafunctional effects.

There must be as much AP space as possible to guarantee a better distribution of forces along and throughout the structure, keeping the cantilever effect to a minimum, or avoiding it altogether, thus facilitating the restoration of a large occlusal surface. This can be achieved by arranging the implants trapezoidally, as much towards the mesial-distal region as possible.

Prosthesis adjustment must be passive to prevent implant fibrointegration.

A fully balanced occlusion is necessary to avoid malocclusion or overlap, which may hinder osseointegration. Centric and eccentric occlusions, both static and dynamic, are balanced occlusions.

7. OSSEOINTEGRATION CONTROL MECHANISM

At present, the best way to measure osseointegration is radiofrequency (Mr Ostell), the benchmark being 60 ISO.

This amounts to monthly periapical x-rays, panoramic x-rays and radiovisiographic images, as well as continuous occlusion monitoring to ensure a balanced occlusion. To assess osseointegration, one must also take into account implant and prosthesis (im) mobility, together with the absence or presence of pain.

The following patient exclusion criteria must be followed:

1. Smokers (more than 15 cigarettes a day)

2. Active periodontal disease:

- 2.a. In the antagonist maxillary bone, which prevents the archival of occlusal stability. Without occlusal stability, the patient will develop occlusal habits which will lead to treatment failure.

- 2.b. Bruxism: The clenching or grinding of the teeth usually overstrains the implants and the temporary prostheses, being capable of causing fractures in the prosthetic restoration, or its displacement, which affects the implants and results in their fibrointegration. To prevent this, dental professionals must be able to assess the diagnostic material correctly.

The remaining teeth and prostheses will help to establish bruxism type and degree, in order to determine whether or not to apply an immediate load.

3. Oral habits:

•Tongue thrust during deglutition

•Typical and atypical deglutition

Both can cause the displacement of the restorative structure.

Considering that the aim of this chapter is to standardize the immediate loading of implants in full mandibular arches, a comprehensive, accurate and accessible classification becomes necessary.

Classification

Six categories have been devised for the purpose:

1. According to their arrangement:

    a-   Intramental

    b-   Behind the mental foramen

2. Implant-assisted immediate loading:

    a-   Modification of prosthetic design

    b-   Necessity

3. According to the surgical technique:

    a-   Implant plus immediate load

    b-   Extraction followed by immediate implant plus immediate load

4. According to the connection type:

    a- External

    b- Internal

5. According to biomechanics:

    a- Full arches

    b- Divided into sections

6. According to the material:

    a-   Acrylic

    b-   Ceramic

7. Due to malpractice

1. According to their arrangement

1a. Intramental:

Implants are placed between mental foramina. This technique is mainly aimed at patients with significant bone resorption in the posterior segment and for prosthetic designs involving no more than ten or twelve teeth and five or six implants. When dealing with replaceable teeth, the status of the antagonist arch, what material to use for the prosthesis and the type of healing process involved must be given careful thought.

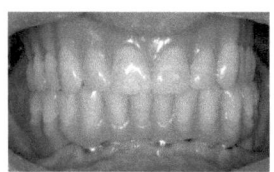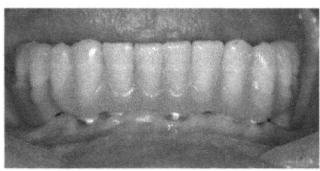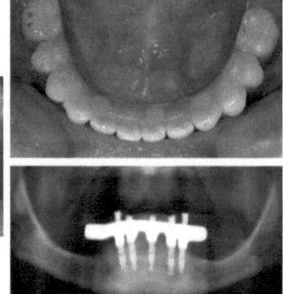

1- Intramental. High complexity hybrid prosthesis .(Mr 3I Osseotite implants)

1b. Behind the mental foramen (postmental):

Advisable in cases with low and even mandibular resorption when compared to alveolar ridge loss, i.e. when there is enough space or bone between the residual ridge and the top of the lower mandibular canal so as to place the implant behind the mandibular nerve. The number of implants will depend exclusively on prosthetic design and on the antagonist arch.

In order to decide whether or not to use the intramental or postmental technique, it is necessary to establish the amount of bone in the residual ridge of the posterior segment with the aim of assessing bone concentration.

Bone stress will depend entirely on the type of occlusion, on the biotype and on the antagonist, which must be considered when choosing a placement technique.

In a study by Dr Vensingol and Dr Weber, published in Joni Vol 10, number 2 (1995), there is a very good description of the biomechanical aspects of two different implant/prosthesis techniques for edentulous patients.

The study concludes that implant arrangement or placement behind the mental foramen enables an optimal distribution of forces. In this case, bone stress will depend exclusively on implant number and arrangement, and on the design and material of the superstructure. The bending strength of the superstructure will greatly influence bone stress concentration.

Therefore, temporary prosthetic structures for immediate loading in full arches must be supported by metallic structures, since the load absorption capacity of acrylic lowers prosthesis utility, the problem with acrylic being that it cannot be divided and, thus, its structure loses strength and is more prone to bending during loading. For this reason, temporary prosthetic structures must be reinforced. Final prosthetic structures must have a metal core, irrespective of whether dealing with medium- or low-complexity hybrid prostheses, with minihybrid ones, or with full crown restoration.

The prosthetic structure must be passive to ensure prosthesis consolidation and avoidance of tensional forces causing bone crest tissue resorption with regard to the implant.

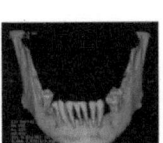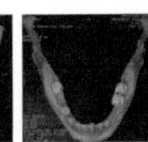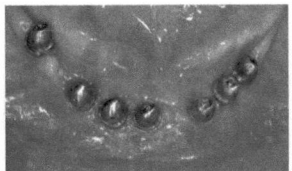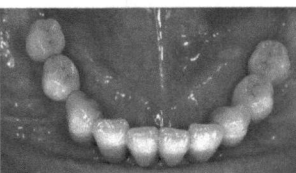

2- Postmental technique. Panoramic view of final restoration High complexity hybrid prosthesis. Titanium Abutments and ten cemented crowns. (Mr 3I Osseotite)

2. Implant – Assisted Immediate Load Implant

2a. Modification of prosthetic design:

It involves changing an already-existing prosthetic design. the prosthetic design of an already-existing overdenture is modified as usual, i.e. going from a removable prosthesis to a hybrid one--classified as a low-, medium- or high-complexity prosthesis (according to the classification suggested by Dr Héctor Álvarez Cantoni)--or to a fixed ceramic prosthesis, depending on facial aesthetics; in other words, on the lip profile resulting from bone loss.

According to a number of surveys, patients are pleased with implant treatment effectiveness, but are displeased with the use of removable prostheses. This appears to be so because they associate implantology with fixed prostheses. At present, it is common to use hybrid prostheses instead of overdentures, since the former are more comfortable and it is easier for the patient to chew, although they are harder to clean and require more maintenance.

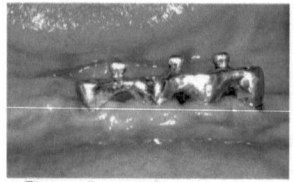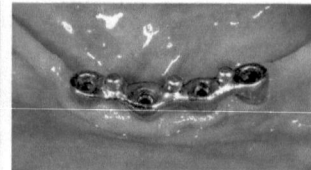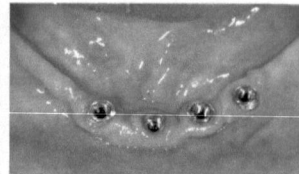

3- Preoperative aspects

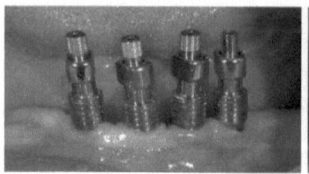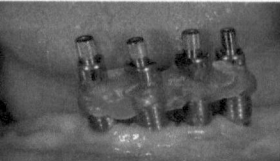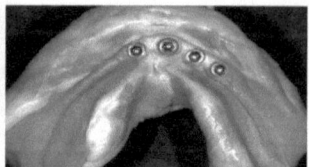

4- Printing existing implants

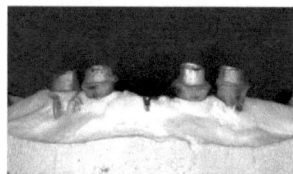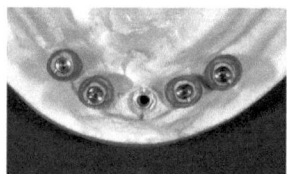

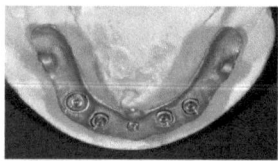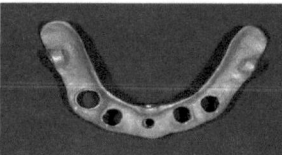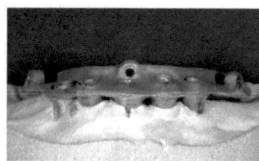

5- Constructing a highly complex hybrid prostheses. With a screw integral with the tray and 4 emerging cemented

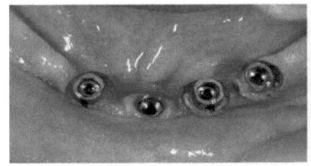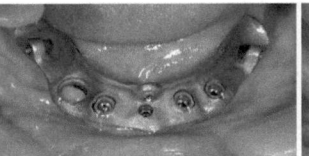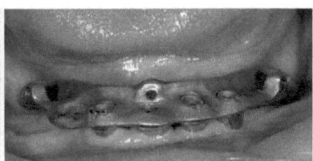

6- Testing passive fit of mesoestructure

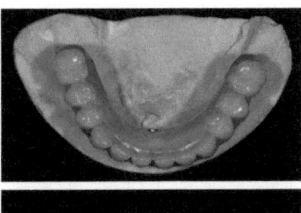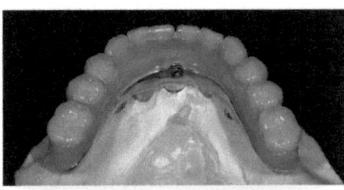

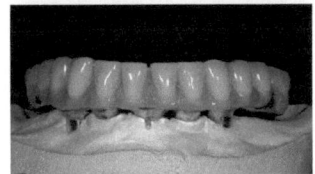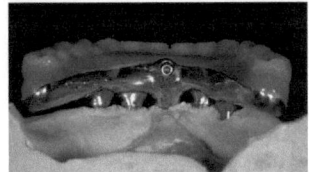

7- Final Restoration

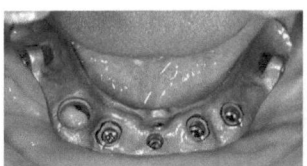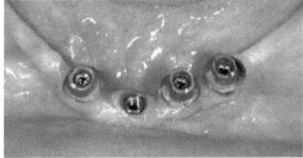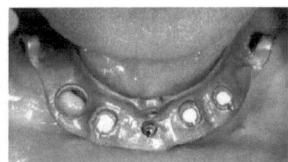

8- Installing the mesostructure and emerging cemented to it

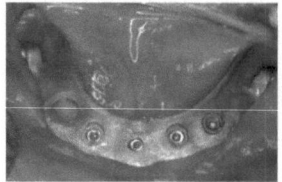 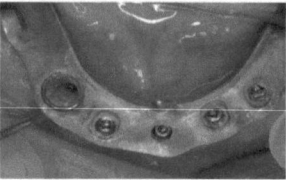 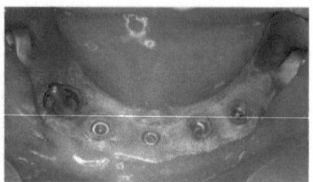

9- Act without surgical incision. Guided by structure Prosthetics

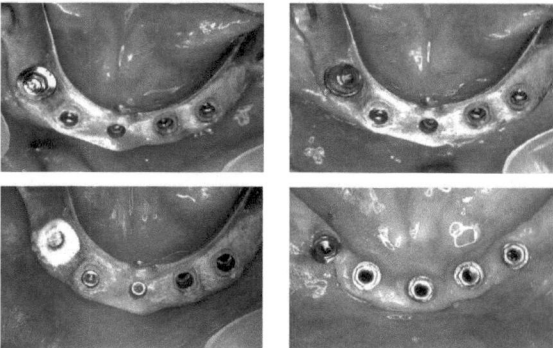

10- Cementation of the mesostructure emerging

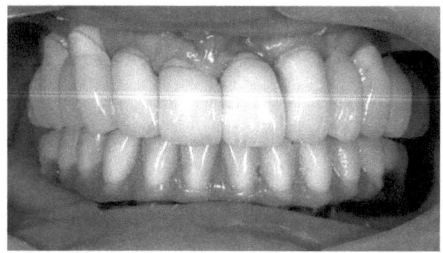 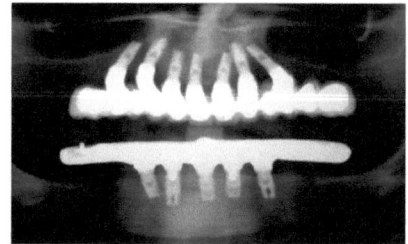

11- Installation of the final restoration

2b. Out of necessity:

Currently, there are different implantology techniques available to answer to a patient's needs, namely the conventional and the two-stage surgical approach in cases in which one of them has failed. Inserting multiple implants in the jaw allows to go ahead with the prosthetic treatment and prosthesis design with a mind to placing or replacing failed implants. This shortens the clinical process, particularly, patient waiting time.

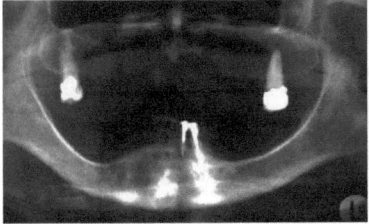
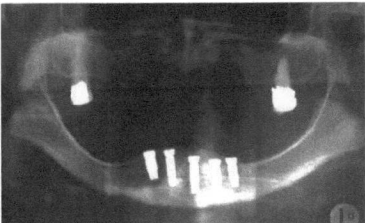

12- Preoperative RX

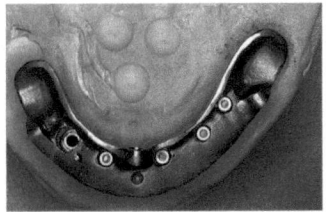
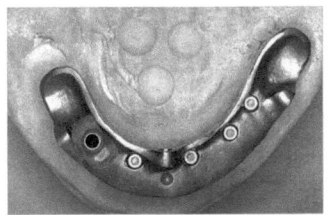

13- Thumbnail mesostructure of highly complex hybrid prosthesis. with surgical guide according to the structure.

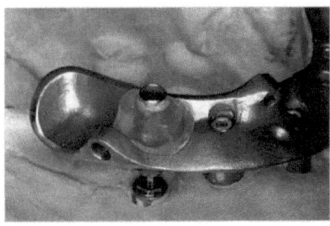
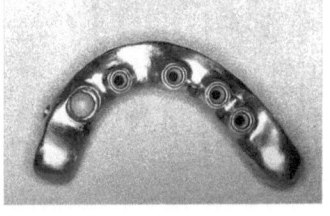

14- Completed mesoestuctura

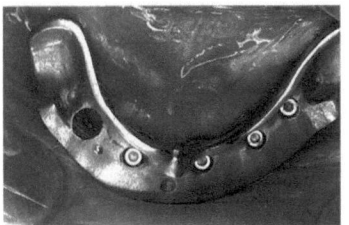
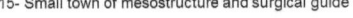
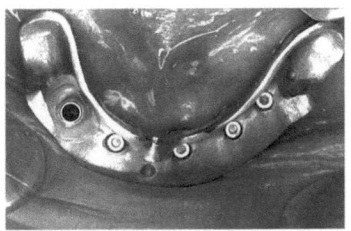

15- Small town of mesostructure and surgical guide

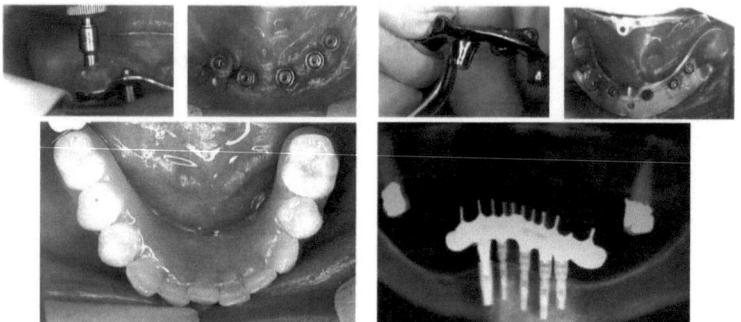

16- Surgery and installation of highly complex hybrid prosthesis. Occlusal view. Rx postoperative panoramic. SIN Implant M.R

3. Surgical Aproach

3a. Implant plus immediate load:

This is the conventional surgical approach, chosen after assessing several clinical x-rays and casts, and based on the patient's bone structure.

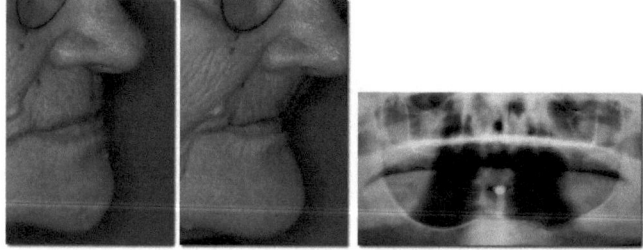

17- Immediate Loading. Patient with prosthesis. Patient without prosthesis. Panoramic rx

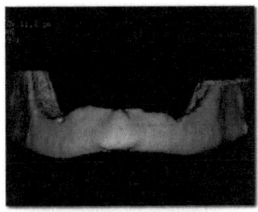
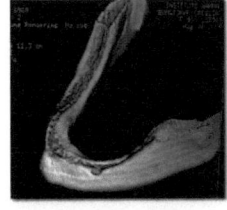
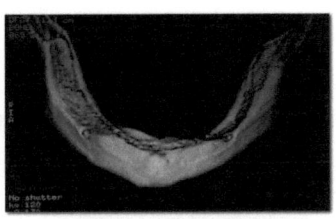
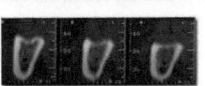
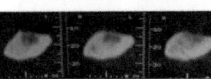
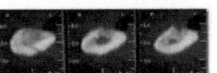

18- 3D ,CAT reconstruction of jaw and Slices CAT of surgical areas

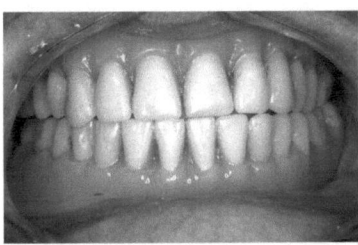
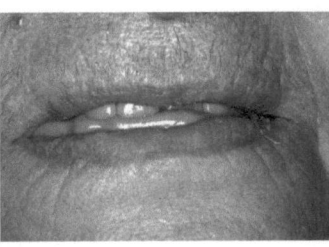
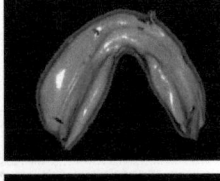
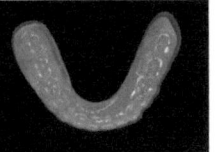

19- Preparation of temporary prosthesis and surgical guide

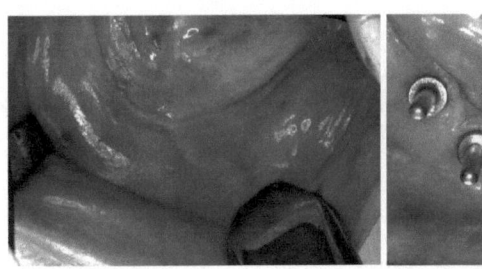
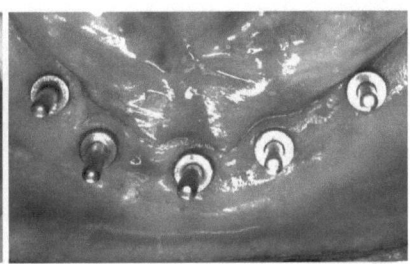

20- Surgery without incision

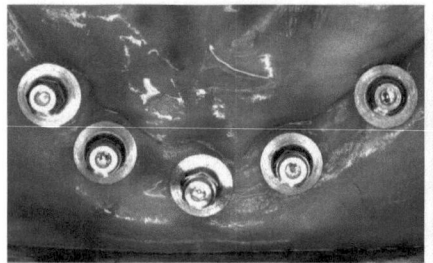
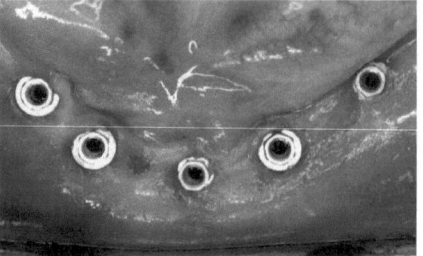

21- Positioning of the implants

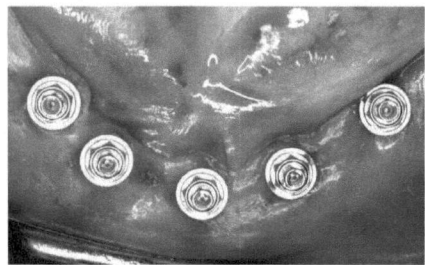
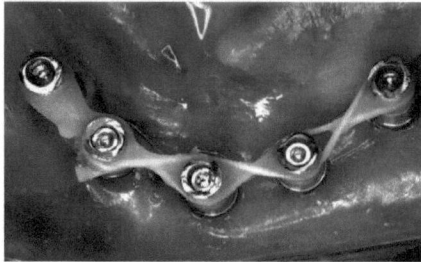

22- Placing and titanium cylinders multiunit

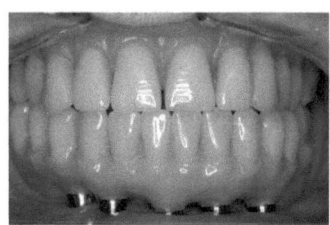
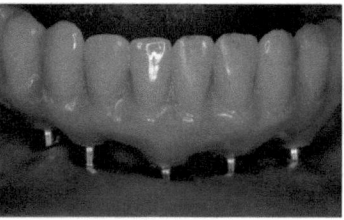
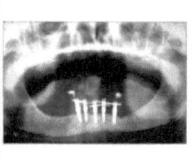

23- Installing the interim hybrid prosthesis and postoperative panoramic rx

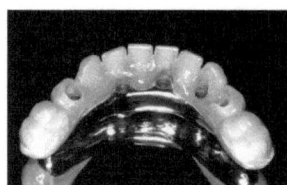
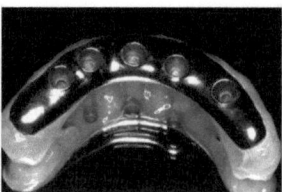
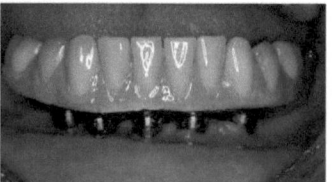

24- Placement of final Prostheses at 3 months

23

3b. Immediate placement of implant after extraction, plus immediate load:

This technique is to be used according to the needs of the patient. It is easier and more efficient because the implant is functional immediately after its placement, which makes it more comfortable and effective than temporary removable prostheses. This method is widely used for patients with the appropriate bone conditions and no infections, which may hinder post-op recovery, such as advanced periodontal disease without active periodontal pockets and cases in which the existing alveolar ridge cannot be used for implant placement, i.e. the alveolar cortical layer will only be used as implant-mandibular ridge anchoring to the bear minimum. Thus, almost 80% will be anchored in the residual ridge of the patient.

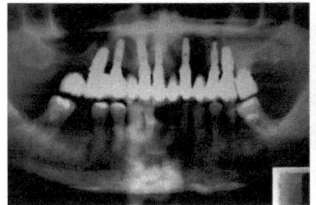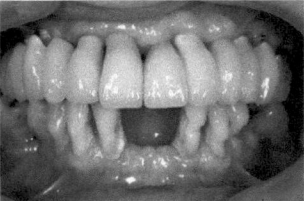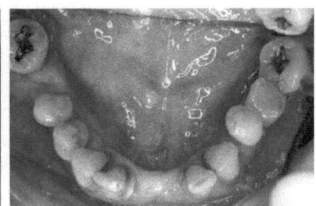

25- Preoperative aspect

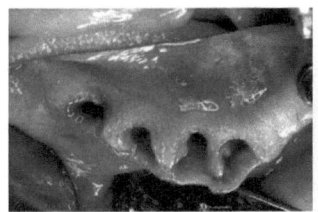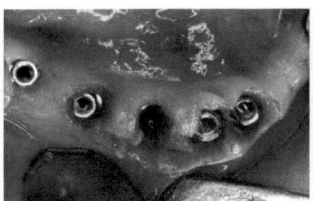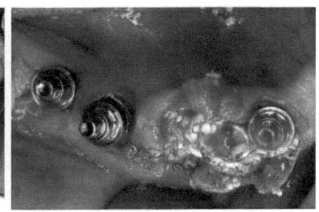

26- Right side. Removal and installation of implants without incision

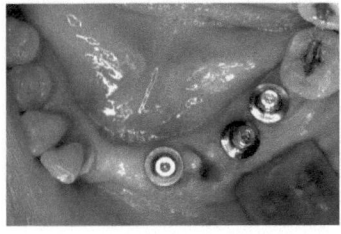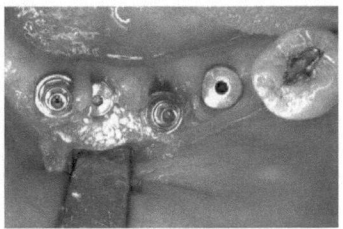

27- Left side. Removal and installation of implants without incision

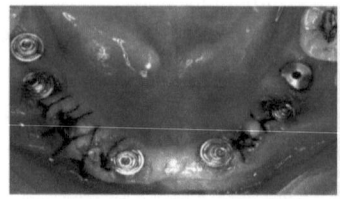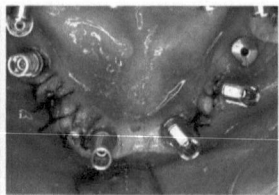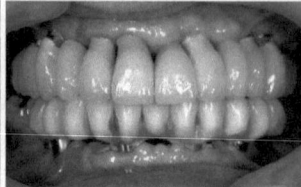

28- Placing titanium cylinders and immediate provisional prosthesis

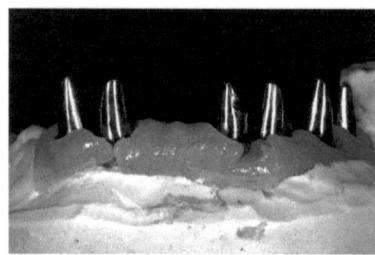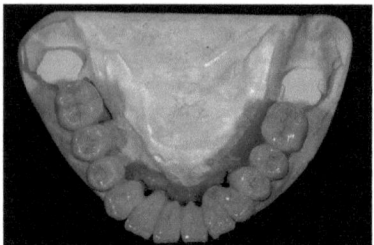

29- Definitive prosthesis. Abutment cuttable and ceramic crowns cemented

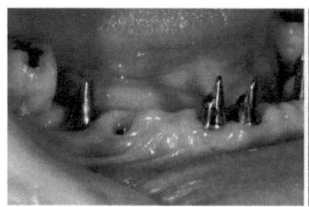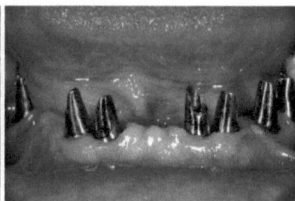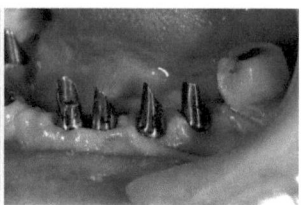

30- Abutment installation

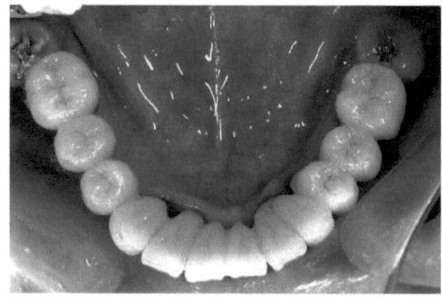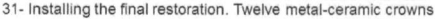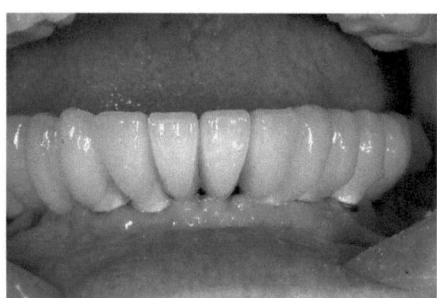

31- Installing the final restoration. Twelve metal-ceramic crowns

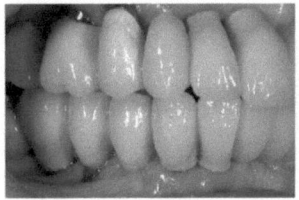 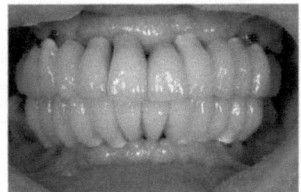 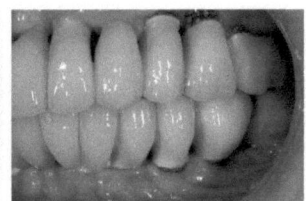

32- Occlusion

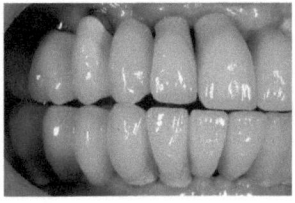 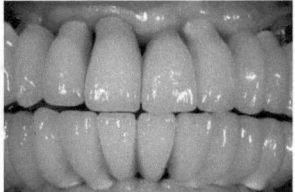 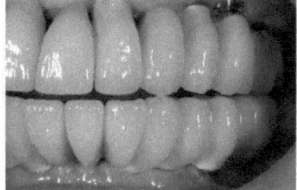

33- Disclusion (propulsion and laterality)

4. Connections

4a. External connection:

It is the most common one. This implantology technique is used in patients having implants with an external hexagon.

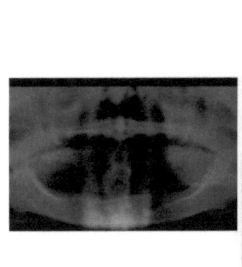 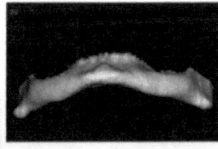 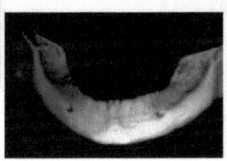 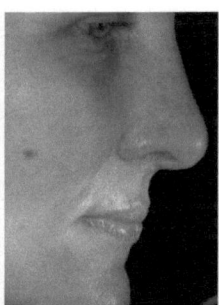 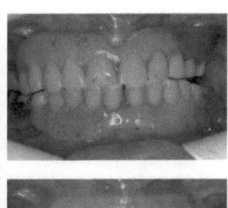 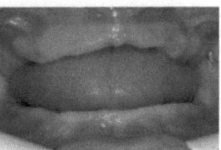

34- External Connection case. Preoperative clinical and radiographic State

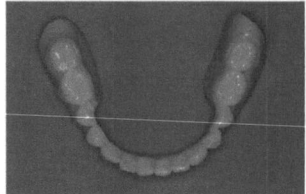

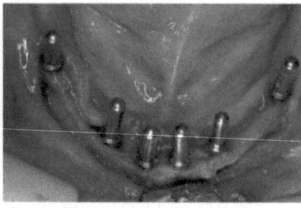

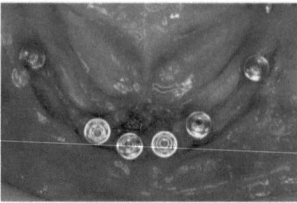

Surgical prosthetic Guide

Surgery. Placement of six implants, four intraforaminales, and two postforaminales (Osseotite 3I).

Conical abutment conection

35

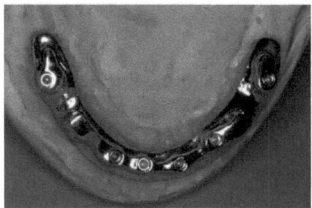

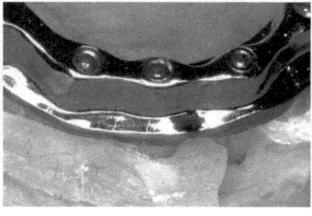

Mesostructure metal casting

Casting superstructure with ceramic pink gum ready to cement twelve pressed ceramic crowns.

36

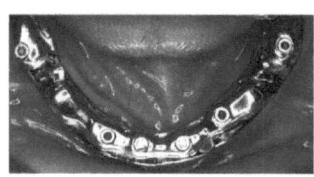

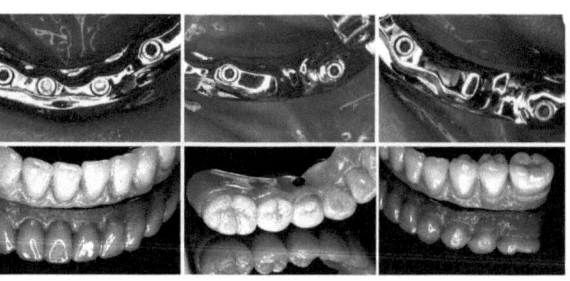

37- Installing Mesostructure

27

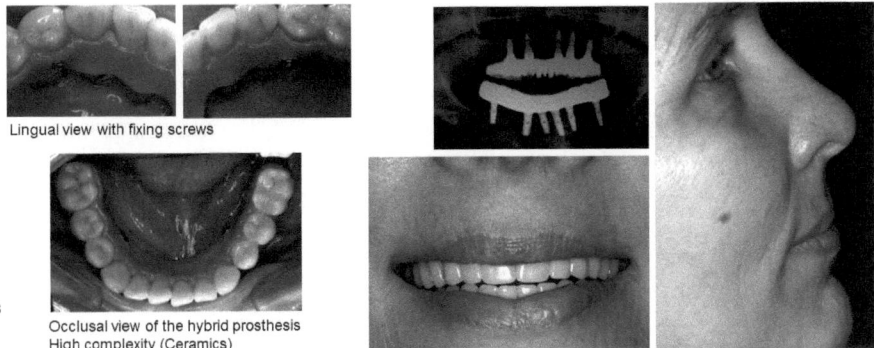

Lingual view with fixing screws

Occlusal view of the hybrid prosthesis
High complexity (Ceramics)

38

4b. Internal connection:

Presently, it is the most popular system due to the fact that the approximation surfaces between the abutment and the implant are much larger, which minimizes any loosening and the creation of gaps.

In turn, it lowers bacteria levels and the risk of peri-implantitis thanks to the use of machined components with approximation surfaces manufactured with computerized alphanumeric drills with a good tolerance range that makes them more accurate than placing cast components against the machined hexagon of the implants, which involves a larger gap and is thus less accurate for adjustment purposes.

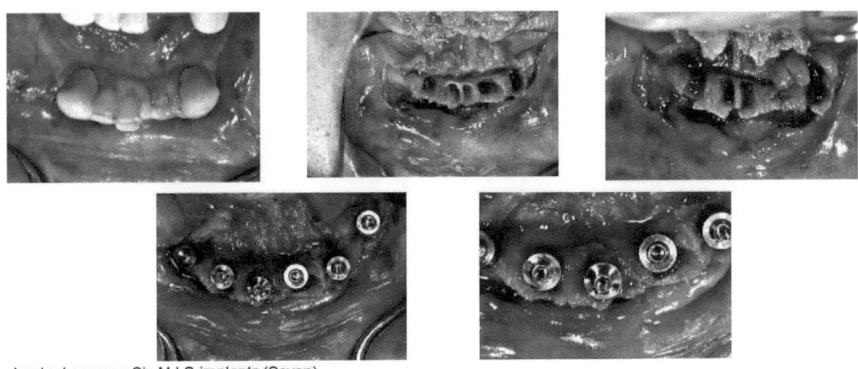

39   Implant surgery. Six M.I.S implants (Seven)

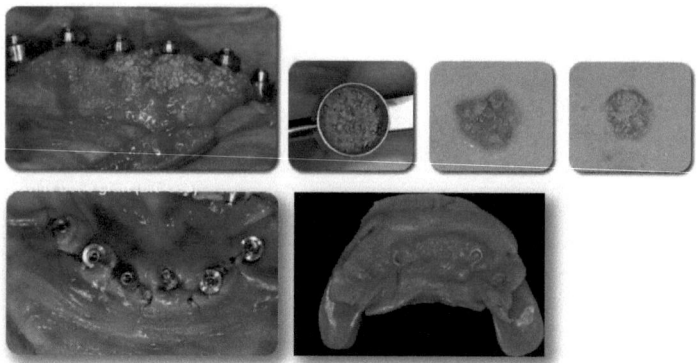

40- Bovine bone graft (Bio-Oss). Placing Multiunit and printing

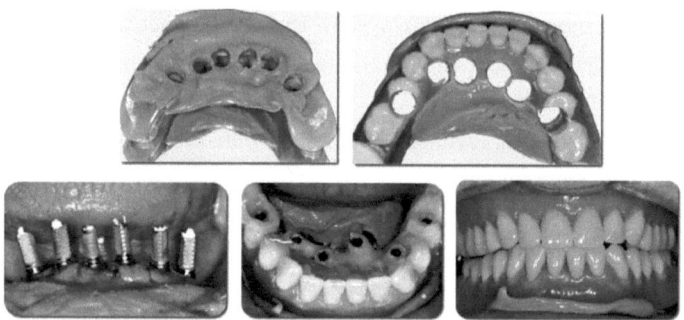

41- Drilling of the provisional prosthesis in the area of the multiunit.
Placing the titanium cylinders, acrylic fixing the prosthesis and check occlusion

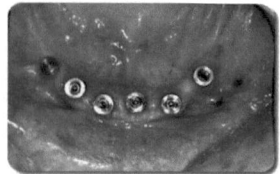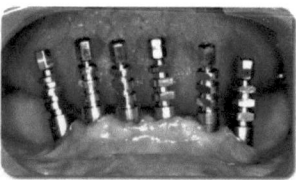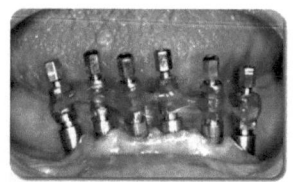

Osseointegration checkup at three months, placement and impression copings splinted them with Triad gel (Dentsply)

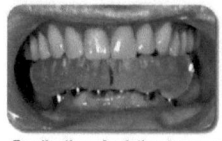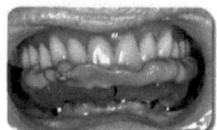

Duplication of existing temporary prosthesis and occlusal registration

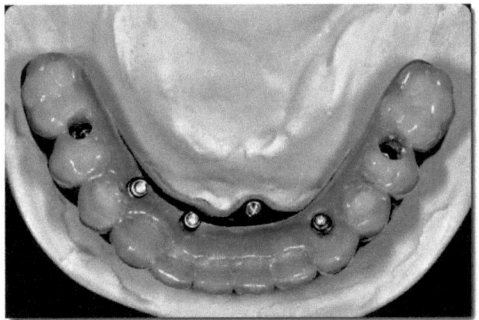

43- Final restoration. Hybrid prosthesis medium complexity

5. According to biomechanics

a- full arches

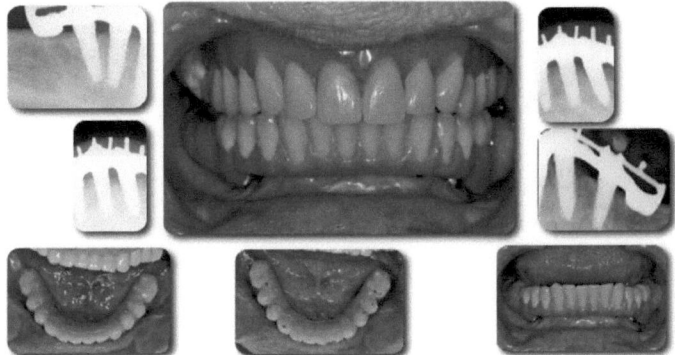

44- Final restoration. Clinical and radiological aspects.

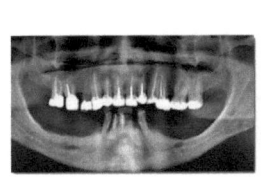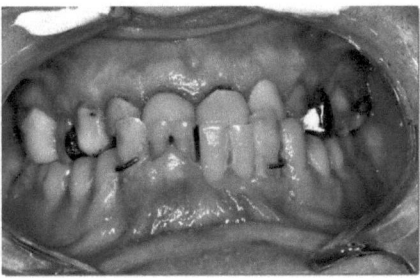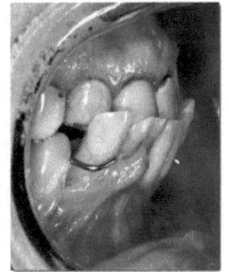

45- Preoperative appearance. Panoramic Rx

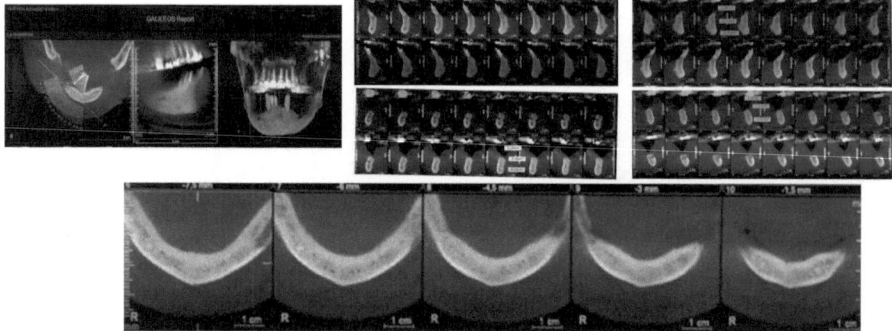

46- Cone beam mandibular

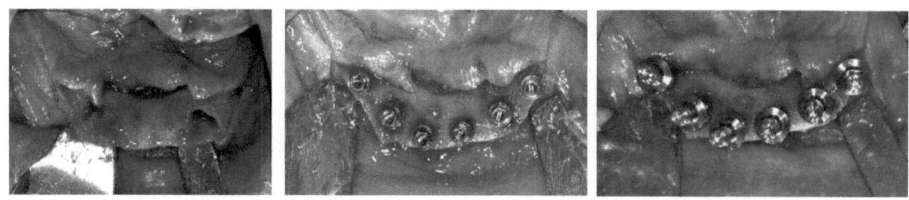

47- Five Implant Placement (Mr 3I Osseotite)

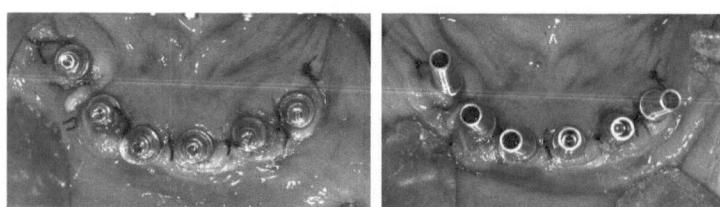

48- Conical abutmen placement and titanium cylinder

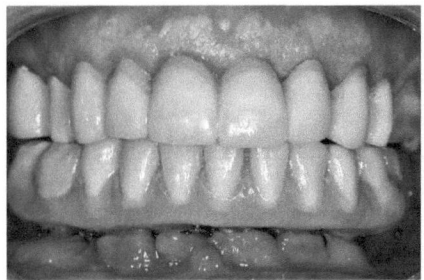 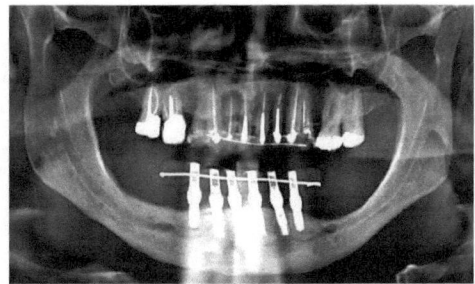

49- Immediate loading with a low complexity hybrid prosthesis and postoperative panoramic rx

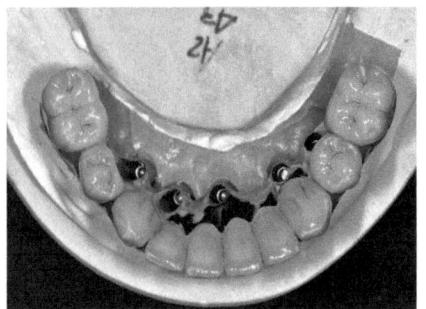 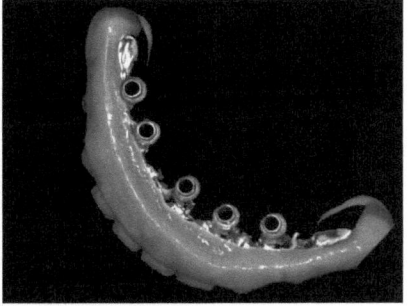

50- Final restoration. Hybrid prosthesis with artificial gingiva

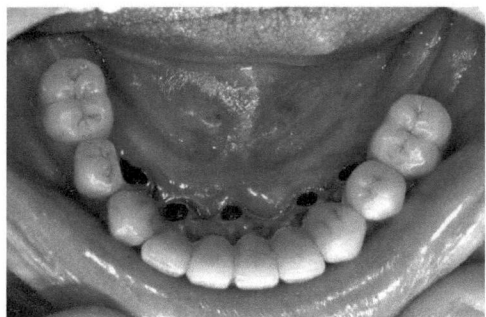

51- Occlusal view

5b. Divided into sections:

Whenever carrying out an immediate load in a full arch, it is necessary to insert a ferule into the structure to generate counterforces in order to stabilize the anteroposterior, lateral, or near-proximal area to achieve a mobility range of less than 100 microns, which the implant needs to achieve osseointegration. After the implant becomes osseointegrated, it can be restored as a full arch with a ferule, or as one divided into sections according to the following elements:

a) Antagonist
b) Occlusion
e) Technical reliability based on implant length

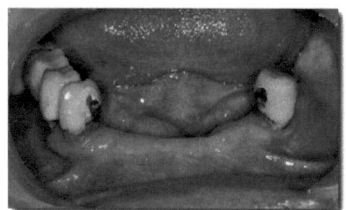 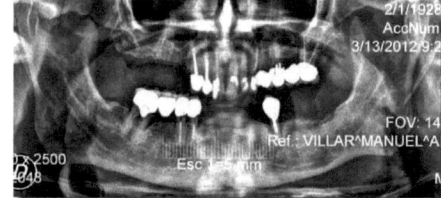

52- Preoperative appearance

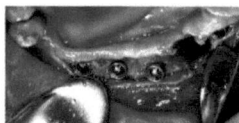 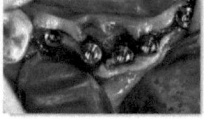 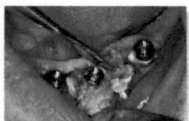 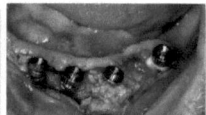

53- Surgery. Eight MIS Implants Placement (seven)

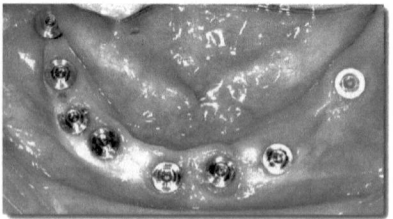 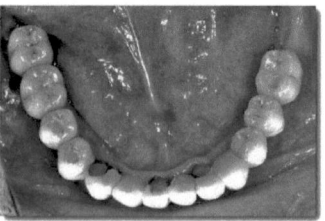

54- Final restoration, screwed and divided into two sections

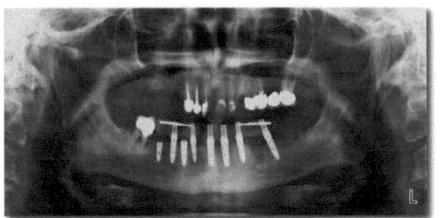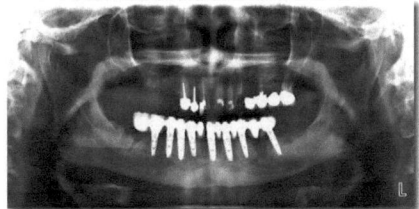

55- Panoramic radiograph post immediately loaded full-arch splinting final divided structures

6. According to the Material

Final restorations may be acrylic, with a hybrid or minihybrid prosthetic design, or ceramic, with a hybrid or minihybrid prosthetic design made entirely out of ceramic. Another viable final restoration method is using ceramic crowns on metal, placing the dental structures directly onto these implants, if able to achieve an aesthetic restoration and a complete bone structure resorption at the level of the dental alveoli. This will require a prosthetic structure for lip support. In this case, hybrid or minihybrid prostheses will be used, always bearing in mind the mesial-distal space needed for stabilization purposes with respect to the antagonist and according to the type of antagonist. Otherwise, the bone resorption, which creates an aesthetic flaw in the prosthetic structure, must be compensated for by means of a full restoration or prosthesis.

a- Acrylic

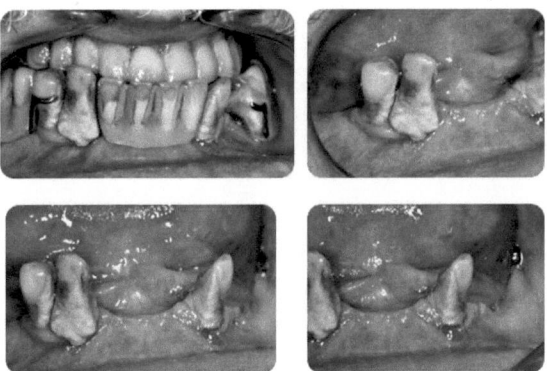

56- Preoperative clinical appearance

34

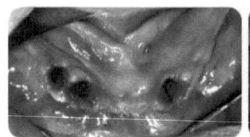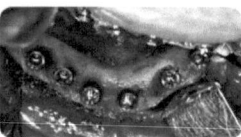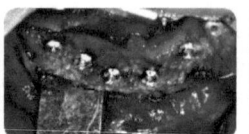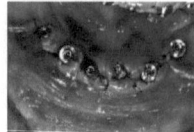

57- Placement of six implants (M.I.S Seven)

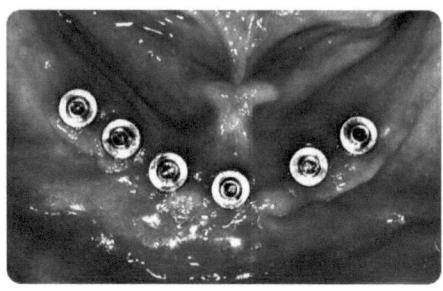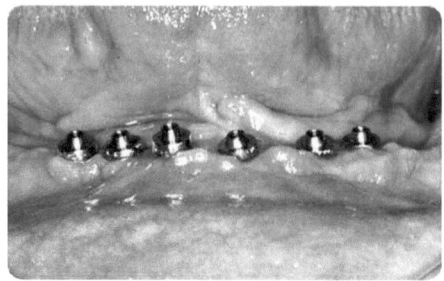

58- Gingival appearance three months after immediate loading

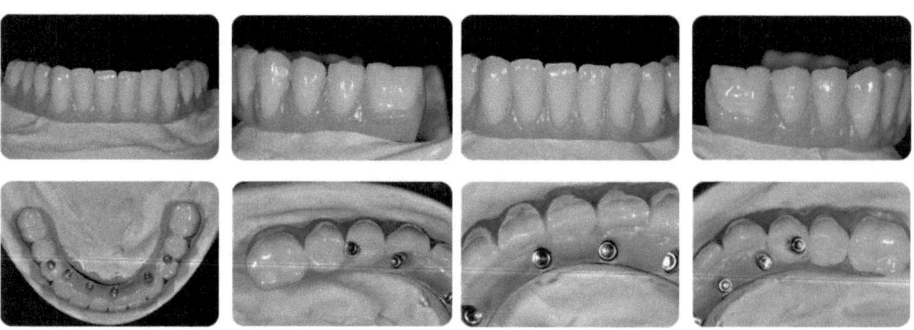

59- Final restoration. Hybrid prosthesis medium complexity

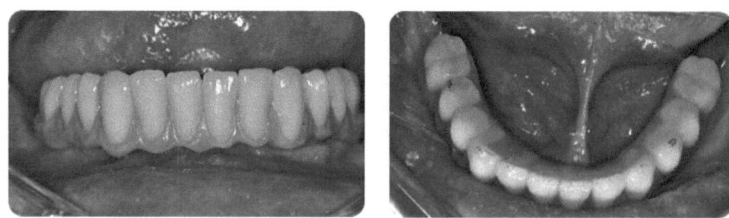

60- Final restoration installed. Buccal and occlusal view

35

b- Ceramic

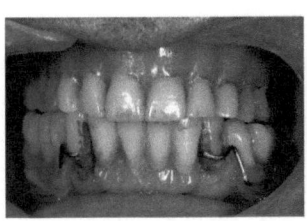
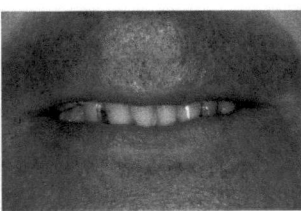
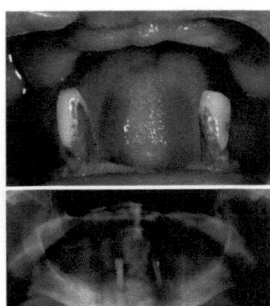

61- Preoperative appearance. panoramic radiograph

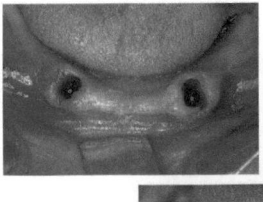
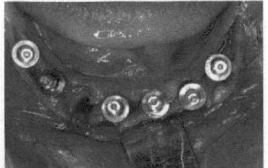
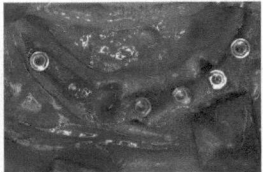

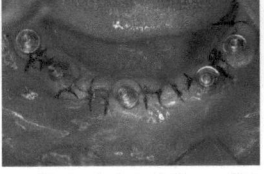
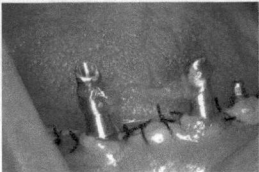
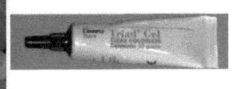

62- Surgery. Six 3i Osseotite implants. Installing and fixing conical abutment with Triad gel (dentsply)

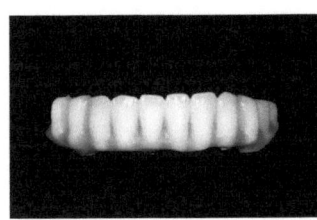
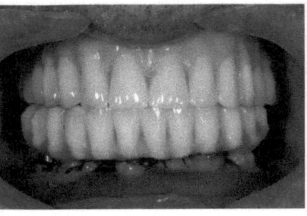
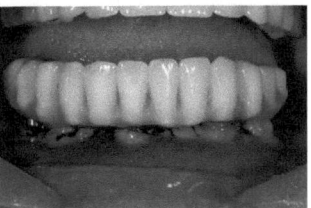

63- Inmediate loading full arch

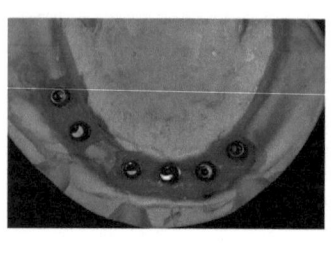
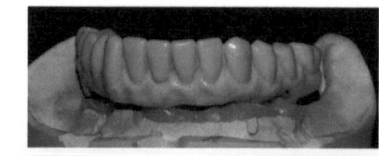
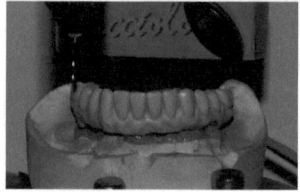
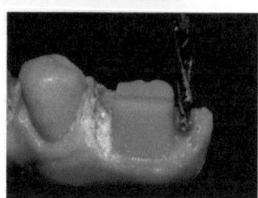

64- Installation six milling abutments and waxing the supraestructure.

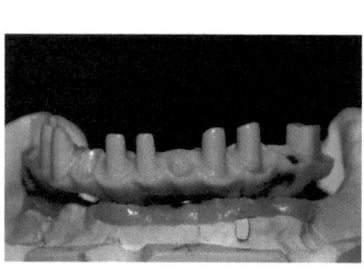
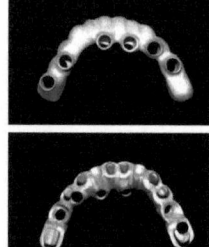
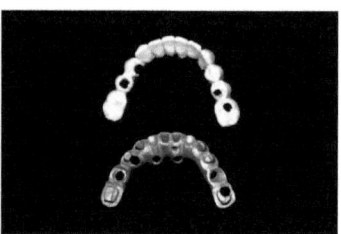

65- Preparation of the metal structure ready to artificial gingiva

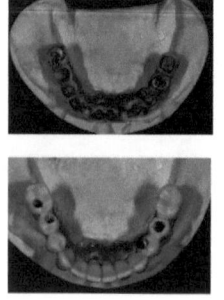
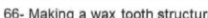
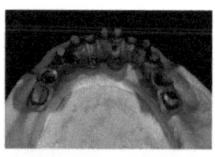
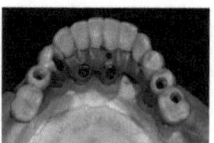
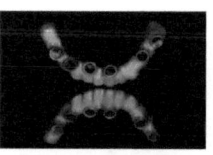
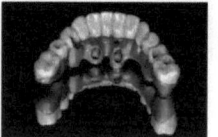
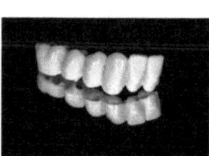
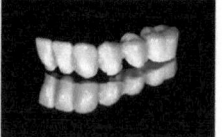

66- Making a wax tooth structure

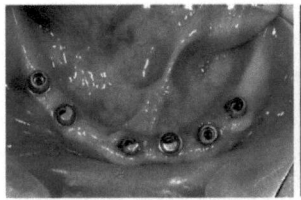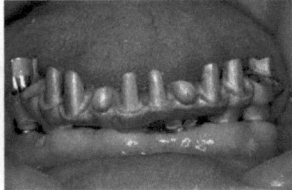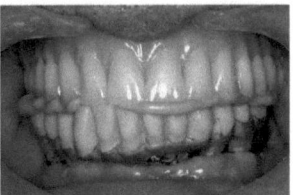

67- Metal control and check occlusion

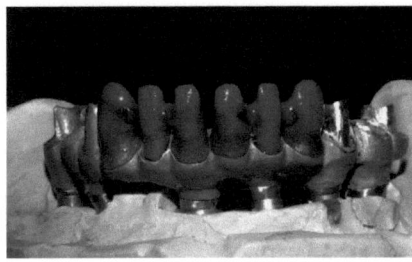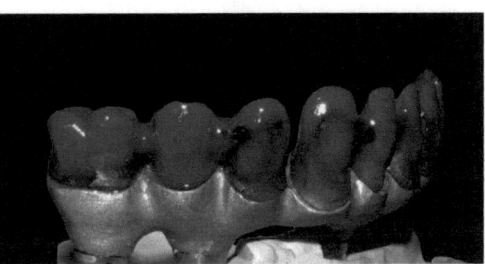

68- Wax structures for making lithium disilicate crowns

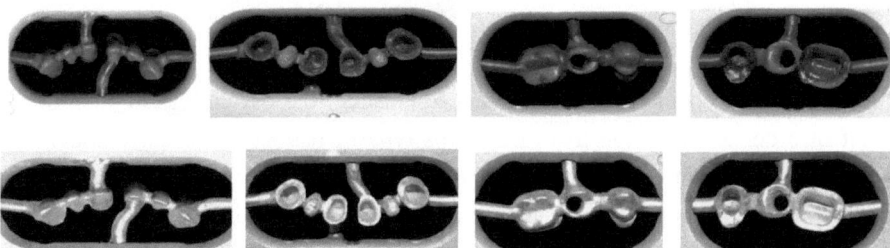

69- Preparation for reading. Sprinkled with silver filings.

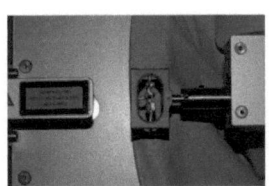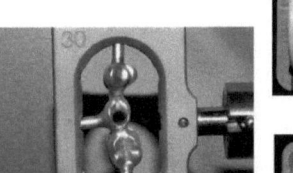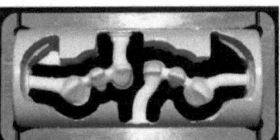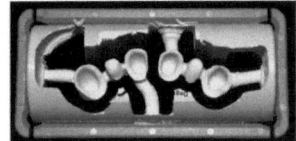

70- Milling with cercom system (dentsply)

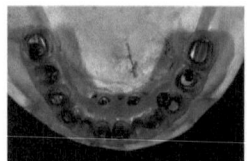
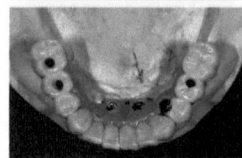
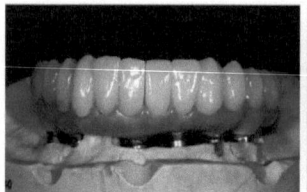
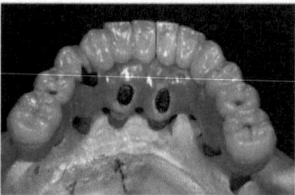

71- Preparation of twelve lithium disilicate crowns modelview

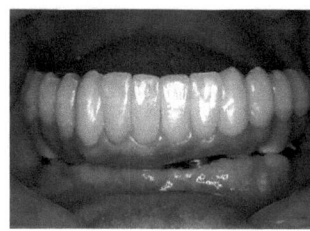
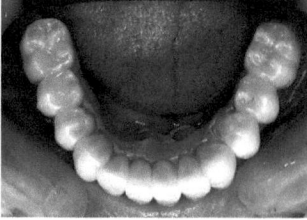

72- Final restoration

7. Due to Malpractice

At this point, it is extremely important to consider the psychological state of the patient in order to apply the treatment. This type of patient has usually undergone implantology procedures which have failed. He or she has most likely been not merely through one, but through many unsuccessful surgeries and, bearing this in mind, clinical treatment time for this procedure is comparatively low.

One final consideration in favor of this treatment is reliability: this technique can be applied in cases in which, in spite of malpractice, there is a high probability of success due to treatment predictability.

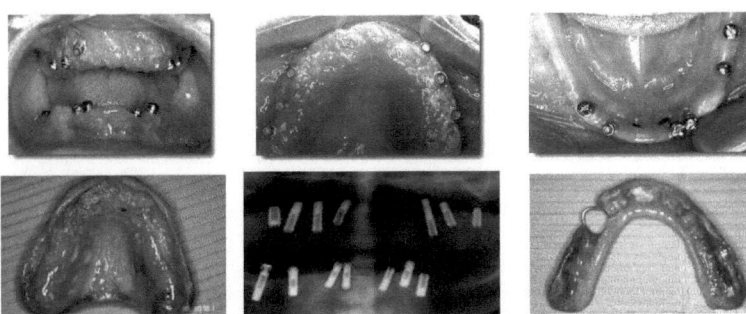

73- Preoperative appearance. Patient with Candidiasis.

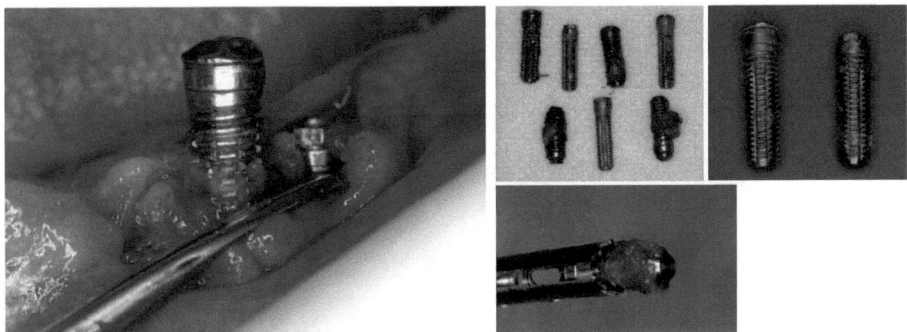

74- Surgical removal of implants

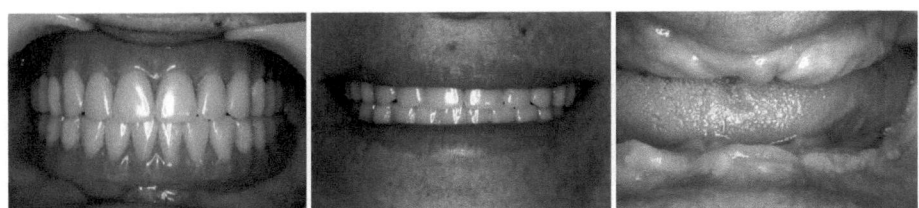

75- Placement of new upper and lower complete dentures

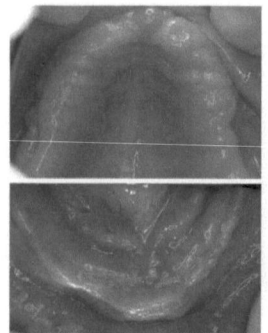
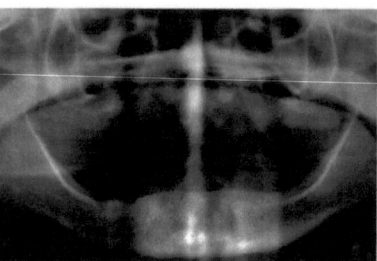
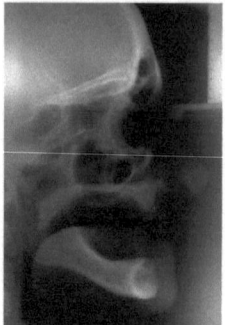

76- Clinical and radiographic appearance 90 days after

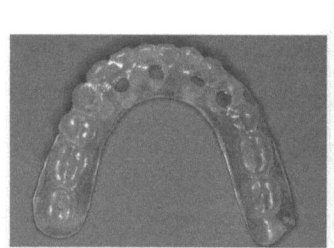
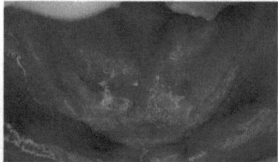
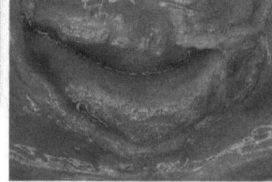
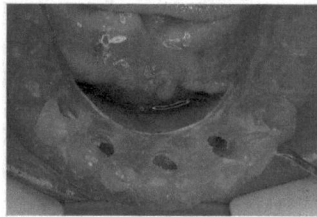

77- Five implant placement with the surgical guide

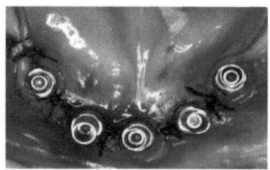
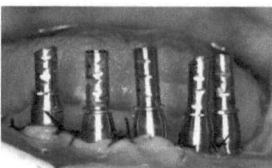
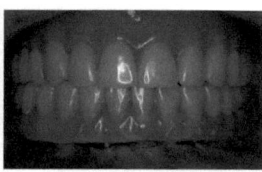

78- Surgery. Five (3I Osseotite implants). Five conical abutments and titanium cylinders and lower hybrid provisional prosthesis

41

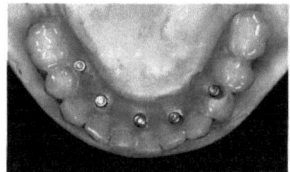
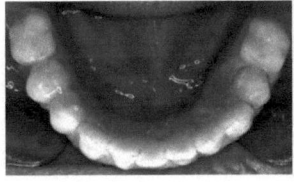
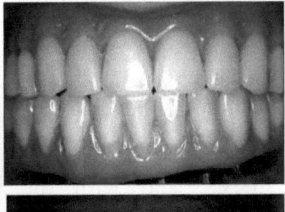
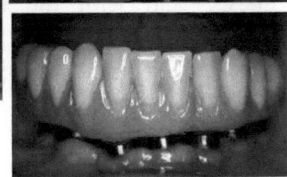

79- Final restoration hybrid prosthesis medium complexity, three months later

Different stages of the technique

There are five:

- *a)* Diagnostic
- *b)* Surgical
- *c)* Temporary prosthesis or osseointegration
- *d)* Gap control
- *e)* Final prosthesis

Having agreed to treat a patient and made a diagnosis, the surgical stage begins: namely, placing the selected implants according to surface and length considerations, following surgical guides and all other appropriate parameters; afterwards, the temporary prosthesis must be inserted. The next stage is one of assessment.

Initially, the patient is examined every seven days in order to check different aspects: firstly, occlusion, so as to maintain centric and eccentric stability; secondly, meso- and suprastructure retention; thirdly, implants, by means of periapical x-rays, RVG or radio-frequency.

Four months after the procedure and according to plan, the final prosthesis is to be manufactured. The prosthetic design will involve either a fixed, porcelain prosthesis on a metal basis, or a hybrid prosthesis. This and occlusion are key elements for maintaining osseointegration.

We have applied this technique at our practice for immediate loading of implants in fully edentulous lower jaws and have developed a standardized protocol that allows us to systematically achieve our goals, from diagnosis to treatment.

Technique Description

Following the diagnosis and treatment selection, we may face different clinical situations: our patients may be fully or partially edentulous, with or without prosthesis, and with the appropriate or inappropriate vertical dimensions or intermaxillary relations.

Consequently, it may prove essential, according to the case and as a complement to the diagnosis, to reestablish the occlusal planes ensuring harmonic vertical dimensions and intermaxillary relations by reliable methods, such as graphic recordings:

> a) Phillips palates
>
> b) Hard palate for central and sole support (BOPAYACU: Spanish acronym)

With a fully functional and aesthetic lower prosthesis as starting point, a self-cured, translucent acrylic duplicate is made by means of a stainless steel muffle, using alginate as duplicating material.

This duplicated prosthesis with orifices can be used as surgical guide for implant placement and for checking that the chimneys have come out properly--these will later be fixed to the temporary hybrid prosthesis. As a secondary use, it can sometimes serve as a guide to create forged or cast metal reinforcements to be used as metal core for the temporary hybrid prosthesis.

Having inserted both the implants and the conical abutments in one surgical action, the connecting chimneys, which have already been cut and tested with the duplicate, are installed and adjusted to prevent them from hindering occlusion when adhering them to the temporary hybrid prosthesis.

Next, using the duplicate as surgical guide, the full prosthesis is trimmed or, if possible, merely perforated for implant placement, taking into consideration the metallic chimneys and taking care not to touch non-surgical areas in order to place them accurately and to enable maximum intercuspation and jaw closing, preserving the stable muscular-skeletal and joint position achieved with a full prosthesis.

The prosthesis is then fixed to the chimneys by means of self-cured, low-shrinkage and rapid polymerization acrylic, until achieving the primary stabilization of all the chimneys.

After polymerizing the acrylic, the chimneys are unscrewed and the prosthesis is removed. It is critical to check that the chimneys are correctly fixed, since the slightest displacement or modification of any of them will prevent the final prosthesis from being perfectly adjusted, a mistake which takes a long time to rectify.

The temporary hybrid prosthesis is to be finished in the laboratory: self-cured pink acrylic must be added gradually, fixing the chimneys and incorporating, if possible, any previously-crafted metal reinforcements next.

The prosthesis must then be trimmed, eliminating the posterior segments, generally the molars, and obtaining a 10-teeth arch. The sides and the lower part are also trimmed, creating convex surfaces separated from the tissue, which enables cleaning. It is important to avoid creating a wide lingual area in order to allow the tongue to move freely, since this is often reported to be uncomfortable and may cause tongue thrusting due to a poor prosthetic design, which hinders implant stabilization and osseointegration.

The prosthesis must be correctly polished and have the appropriate finish to prevent the surface from retaining large amounts of bacteria and to prevent the prosthesis from irritating the mucous membrane.

Once finished, the prosthesis must be fitted in the patient's mouth, checking for correct placement and adjusting the occlusal microscrews linking the chimneys and the conical abutments.

The final steps are checking that the jaw closes properly and adjusting centric and eccentric occlusion, so that it is organic and safe, which should not be difficult if the position achieved when fixing the prosthesis to the chimneys has been preserved. The chimneys are then covered with light-curing, resilient resin.

The patient will go back to his/her everyday life, being essential for him/her to mind his/her eating habits and oral hygiene, as well as to undergo the necessary checks and controls.

Seven days after surgery, the sutures must be taken off and hygiene and occlusion checked.

It is advisable to undergo frequent clinical-radiographic examinations until osseointegration is achieved.

Final Prosthesis

Having achieved osseointegration, the temporary hybrid prosthesis can be easily and rapidly removed by taking off the well-preserved resin plugs and the occlusal microscrews.

If the patient's hygiene has been good, the peri-implant gum should be in perfect condition.

This clinical and radiographic examination is critical, since after corroborating implant osseointegration, a cast of the implants and an intermaxillary recording can be made, which will help to manufacture the final prosthesis.

Afterwards, either impression transfers or copings must be chosen for the conical abutments, adjusting the screws onto them.

It is a good idea to tie them with dental floss, which will serve as scaffolding for the low-shrinking acrylic that acts as a ferule for the impression transfers or copings.

The acrylic must be skillfully manipulated to minimize shrinking, which although low, does always take place. It is advisable to cover the transfers first and, once polymerized, to bind them with acrylic bridges.

This splinting system keeps them stable and enables a very accurate adjustment of the metallic structure of the future prosthesis, if the metallic material is manipulated properly.

An impression is obtained at once with heavy silicone fluid, using a perforated tray and regular silicone or silicone fluid. This implant and conical abutment position transfer technique is achieved through transfer dragging.

Reproducing the peri-implant tissue accurately is crucial for the prosthetic design to enable hygiene.

While the impressions are being taken, a trained assistant can easily duplicate the temporary hybrid prosthesis in the laboratory with the same technique used to duplicate the full prosthesis.

Having obtained a duplicate, it must be placed on the conical abutments, checking for stability and appropriate lodging after minor adjustments. Next, vertical dimension and occlusion must be checked, using the initial temporary prosthesis as reference.

This step greatly simplifies the procedure, saving time (less visits to the dentist) and allowing the duplication, maintenance and transfer of the prosthetic area, and of the dimensions and relationships achieved at the point of departure by means of accurate techniques.

Once a duplicate has been achieved, an intermaxillary recording must be made with silicone, which will help to set up the working casts correctly.

The temporary prosthesis must then be inserted and the impressions and recordings sent to a dental technician.

In the next visit, the final prosthesis must be tested according to its type.

Normally, the testing of medium- or high-complexity hybrid prosthesis involves checking the metallic structure and teeth alignment. The metallic structures can be adjusted easily and accurately thanks to the nature of the aforementioned impression methods, to the availability of cutting-edge materials and to the manufacturing techniques applied by highly-specialized dental technicians.

If the treatment includes crown rehabilitation, the metallic structures have to be tested and the color chosen, since it must be the same both for the stock teeth and for the ceramic guide.

The following visit must be aimed at finishing the final prosthesis. It must be retested, checking for good adjustment and occlusion—please note that placement procedures vary according to prosthetic type.

If working with a low-complexity hybrid prosthesis, it must be fixed with occlusal microscrews and the chimneys must be covered with a Teflon plug for protection purposes, placing a composite plug over the latter. In the case of high-complexity hybrid prostheses, the abutments must be screwed and fixed with resin cement to the suprastructure, set in place while screwing the auxiliary abutment. After polymerizing the cement, the entire structure is to be removed and any protrusions trimmed and filed. The prosthesis must be fitted for the last time and the upper part of the suprastructure containing the teeth and gum must be sealed and screwed in.

If the final prosthesis includes porcelain crowns, the abutments must be inserted first. Then, the crowns must be microscrewed onto them and cemented. For cemented structures, it is best to create small holes in the lingual-crown chimney area in case it should be necessary, at some point, to enlarge them or to reach the screws.

A final occlusal adjustment must be made to ensure an organic and safe occlusion, and the patient must be given, once again, hygiene and maintenance instructions.

It is advisable for the first check-up to take place one week afterwards, at which time an organic safety plate should be ideally installed, therefore ending the prosthesis manufacturing and placement process, and discharging the patient.

Further check-ups must be scheduled as necessary, bearing in mind important factors such as hygiene, bruxism, occlusion and antagonist type. Thus, the examinations may take place monthly, every three months, once or twice a year.

Clinical Case

After becoming familiar with the different stages of the technique, and having understood them, one is faced with variables stemming from technological advances, which have modified immediate loading success parameters, making it routine and predictable. In turn, these require new techniques that become easy-to-apply protocols conducive to lowering the clinical time of the procedure, facilitating the work of the professional and increasing patient comfort, which leads to a better postoperative.

At present, we rely on four standard techniques, depending on the clinical case:

1- Pick up Technique

2- Peek abutment technique

3- Impression technique

4- Stereolitographic model technique

Pick up Technique

This technique was developed 10 years ago by Dr Galucci and it consists of determining occlusal parameters and vertical dimension during the planning stage, making a temporary structure to be duplicated in order to enable the placement of the prosthetically-guided implants. This will be then fixed to the implants on the basis of the selected components.

The right finish is later achieved in the laboratory.

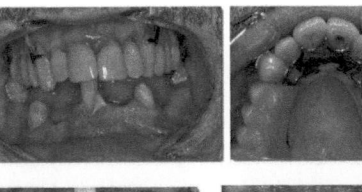
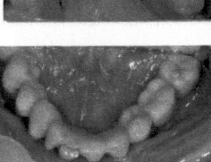
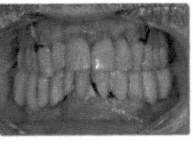
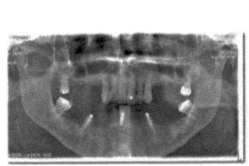
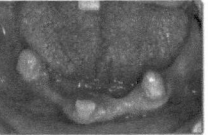

80- Preoperative picture and panoramic Rx

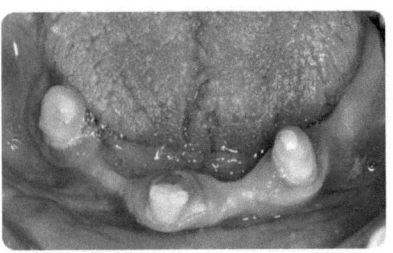
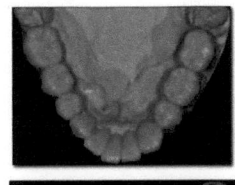
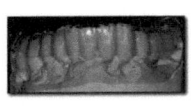
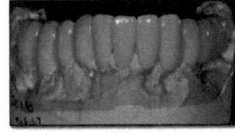
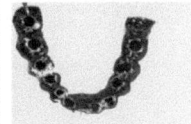

81- Twelve making temporary crowns and a surgical guide

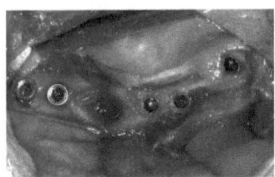
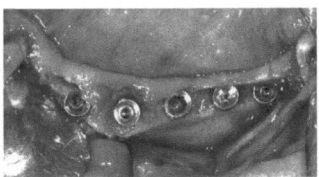
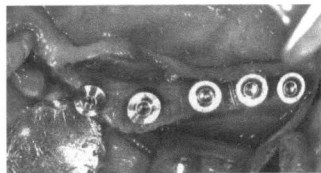

82- Surgery. Teen placement Seven implants (MIS) and multiunit components

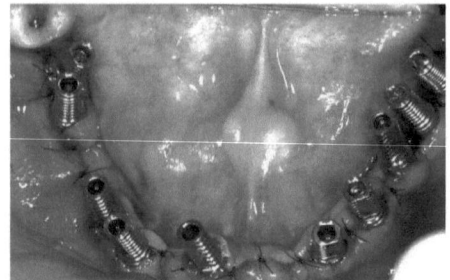

83- Placing titanium cylinders

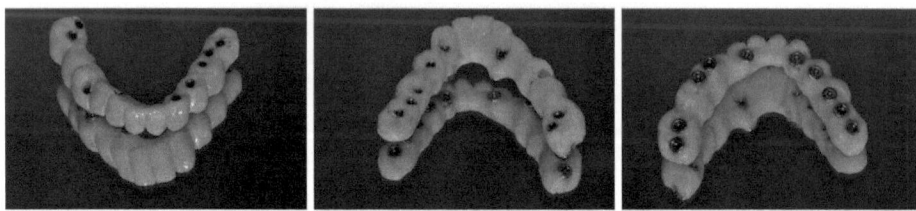

84- After titanium cylinders placed trails with the interim

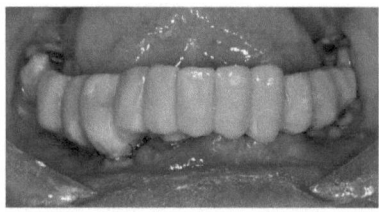

85- Installing interim Rx screwed and postoperative

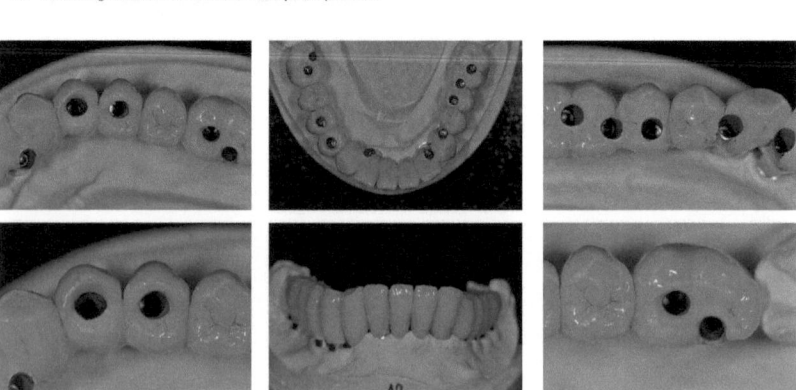

86- Final restoration. Twelve metal-ceramic crowns screwed

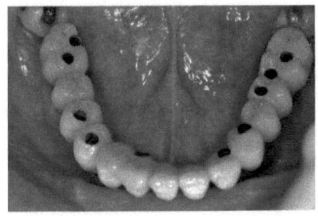 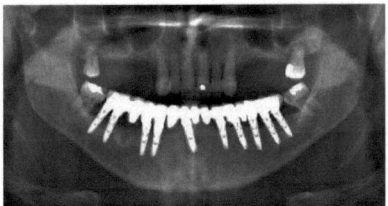

87- Final restoration. Postoperative panoramic radiograph

Peek abutment Technique

Tecapeek TM is an ultra light, thermoplastic, biocompatible, high-performance polymer (polyaryletherketone), both hard and stiff. Regarded as ideal for medical applications, it is aimed at supporting structures. The subtype used in medicine is known as Tecapeek Classix TM.

Production Techniques:

      1. Injection molding

      2. Machining

      3. Compression molding

Properties:

1. High mechanical strength and chemical resistance, ensuring dimensional stability

2. Good wear resistance for manipulation purposes

3. Good impact and abrasion resistance

4. Easily sterilized (autoclave, gamma radiation, ethylene oxide) without affecting its mechanical properties

5. Good high-temperature and hydrolysis resistance

6. The product can be made to have extremely thin walls due to the mechanical properties of the material, which is structurally stiff

7. Standard colors: white and beige

Specifications:

The material is FDA-approved for medical applications, being biocompatible with tissue and free of cytotoxicity. It is also ISO 10993 certified.

This material can be in contact with blood and tissue for 30 days and tests are being carried out to determine whether extended use can lead to any side-effects.

Medical Applications and Techniques

1. Tubes, catheters, laparoscopes, endoscopes, and other wire-type devices

2. Devices in contact with blood (dialysis)

3. Temporary dental implants

4. Generally used in neurology, urology, gynecology and the pharmaceutical industry

In the field of dentistry, this type of abutment is used routinely for the following:

a- Immediate loading

b- Immediate prosthesis

c- Second stage surgery

Immediate loading and prosthesis are standard techniques requiring abutment. In the case of immediate loading, this is aimed at creating a prosthetic structure capable of withstanding the loading procedure while enabling normal osseointegration and soft tissue restoration.

In connection with immediate prostheses, the material facilitates the creation of a temporary structure without resorting to loading, its function being to maintain and restore the patient's gingival structure by shaping the biological width and preserving the esthetic aspect

As regards second stage surgery, previously known as "aperture," it has gained great importance in the sector for its esthetic and biological advantages: it contributes to preserving gingival esthetics and peri-implant health, offering stability and durability.

With the introduction of the Tecapeek TM abutment into the market, temporary abutments were simplified:

1. Easy to drill

2. Non-toxic

3. Leaves no residues in soft tissue after manipulation

4. Can be in contact with blood or fluids for 30 days (FDA recommendation); in fact, at our practice, we have used it for 3 months for immediate loads and prostheses without recording any structural problems: it withstands occlusal loads with very little imbibition and, thus, it does not lose its shape

5. For temporary restoration, the implant can be attached with a temporary or permanent luting agent without compromising its structural integrity

6. Available in the market for external and internal connection of 3I and Biohorizons implants, manufactured by various companies (3I, Bihorizons, Q Implant, M.I.S)

Being easy to manipulate and remaining cool during drilling, its mechanical strength allows for angle correction without compromising structural integrity; additionally, since it remains stable over time, it can be in contact with soft tissue safely for a long period, allowing to shape the biological width. The alignment between implant and abutment is very good.

From a clinical standpoint, this moderately-priced method accelerates and simplifies treatment, for which it is widely used today.

Clinical cases

First case.

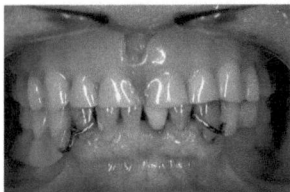 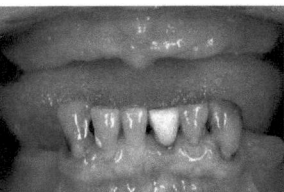 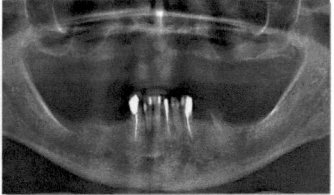

88- Preoperative appearance. Panoramic Radiography.

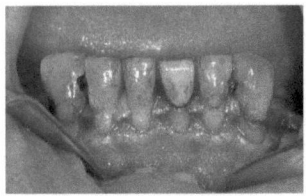 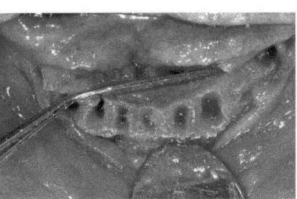 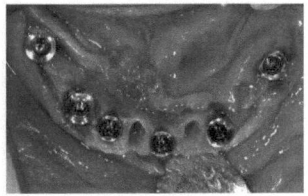

89- Extraction of the remaining teeth and bone flattening placement of six implants (3I Mr Osseotite)

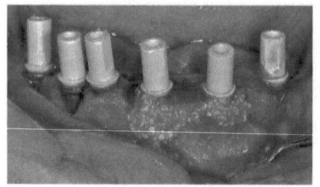
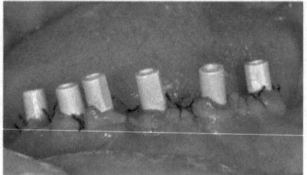
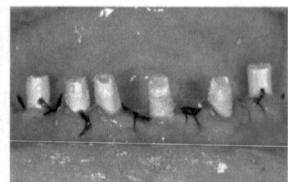

90- Peek abutment placement Q-implant

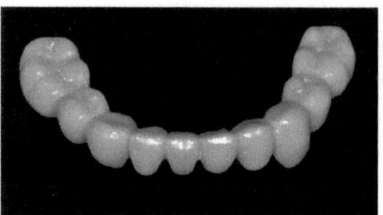
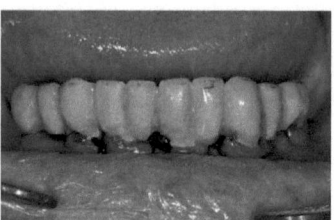

91- Cemented fixed prosthesis

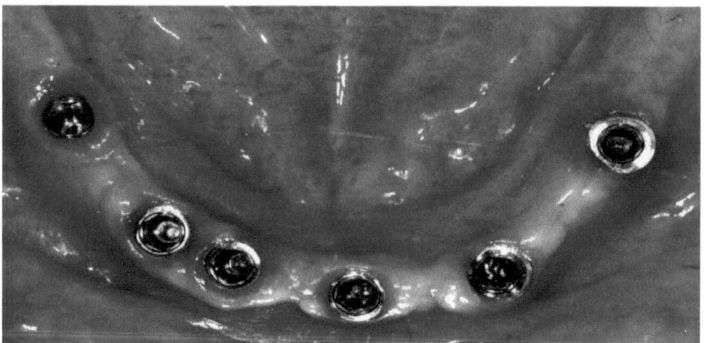

92- Clinical aspect three months later

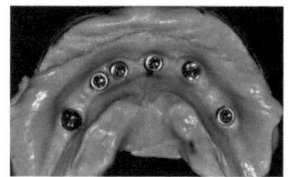
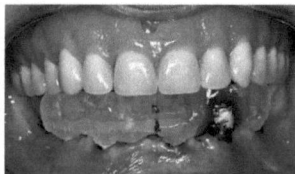
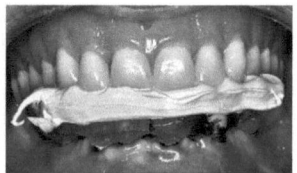

93- Pull printing and duplication of provisional restoration

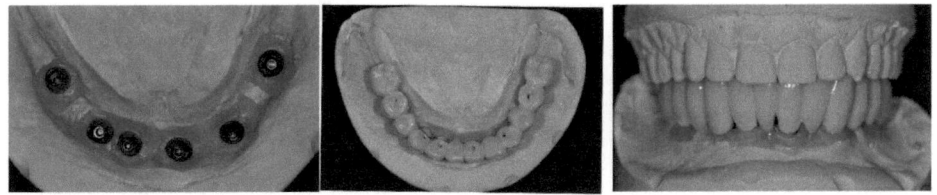

94- Prosthetic Restoration. Abutment carvings. cemented crowns

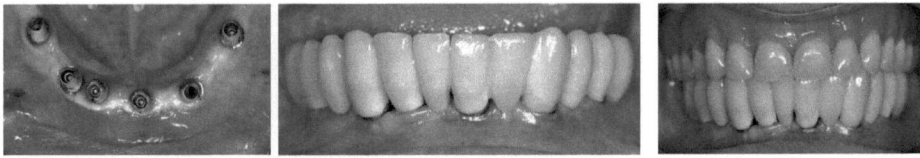

95- Final restoration. Twelve cemented crowns

Second case

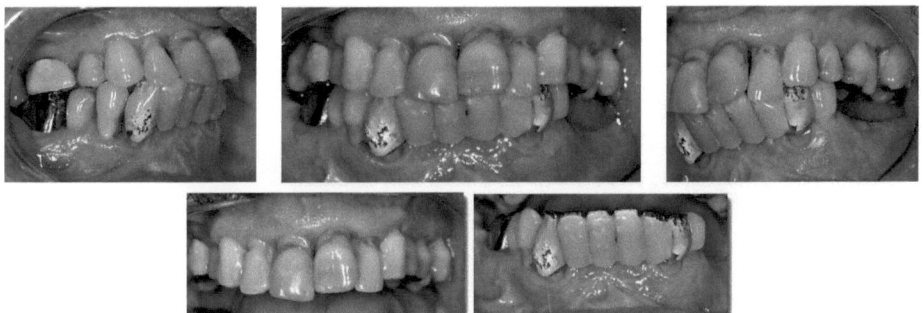

96- Preoperative appearance

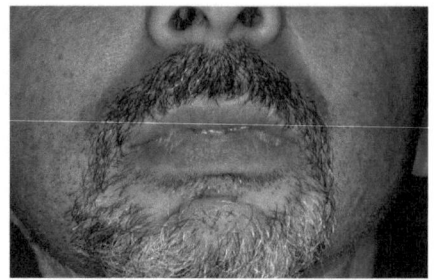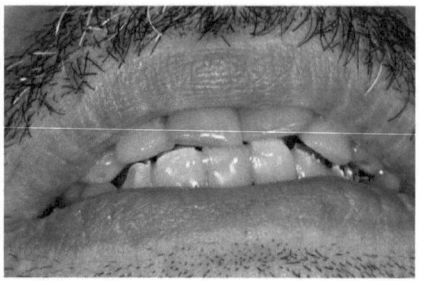

97- Facial appearance

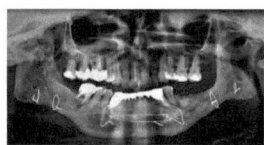

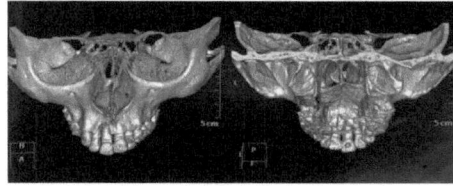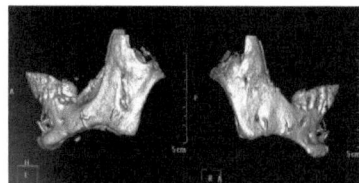

98- Panoramic Rx and Tomography

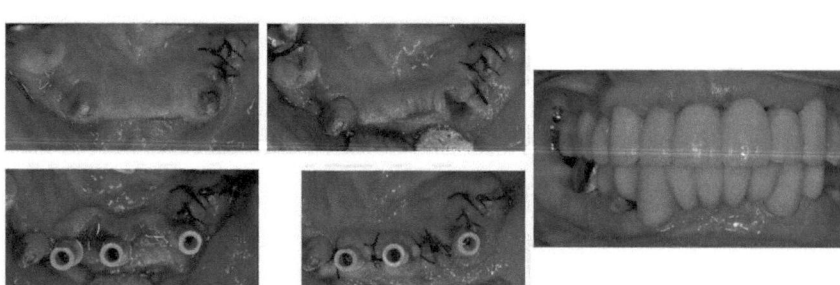

99- Surgery. Five 3i-Osseotite certain implants peek abutment and inmediate loading

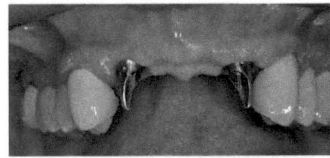

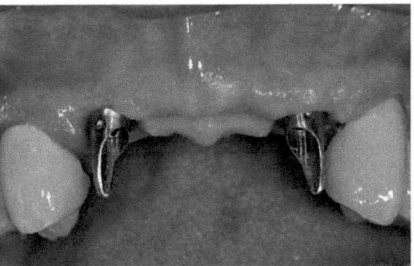

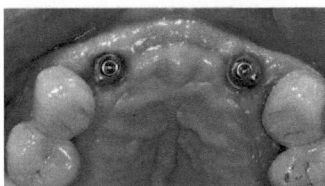

100- Final restoration. Abutment installation

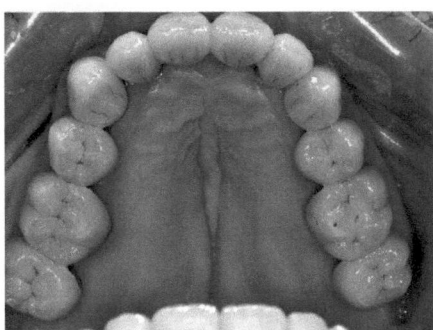

101- Final restoration. Occlusal view

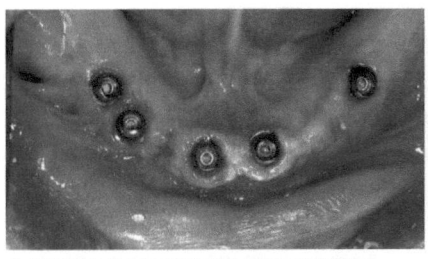

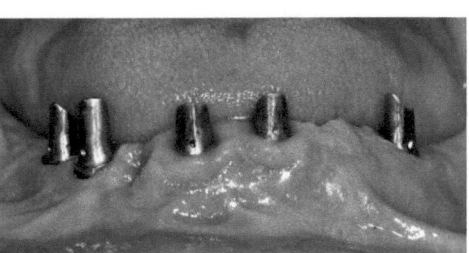

102- Mandible. Abutment installation three months later

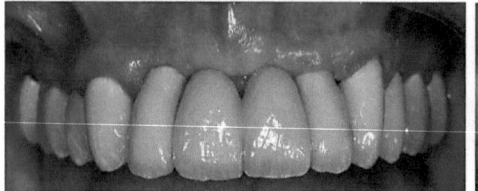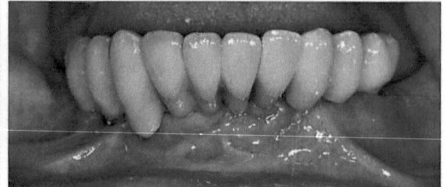

103- Vestibular view. Upper and lower. Final restoration

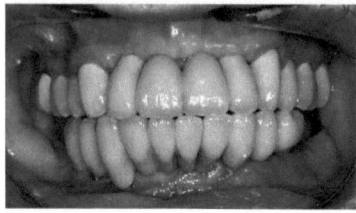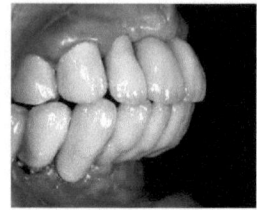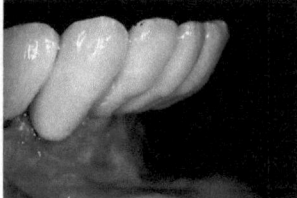

104- Occlusion and lateral view

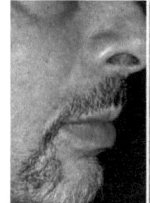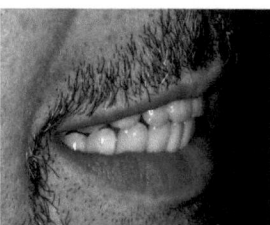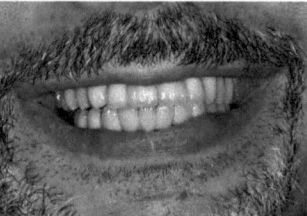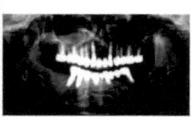

105- Final facial appearance. Postoperative Panoramic Rx

Impression Technique

In this case, following implant placement, the appropriate prosthetic components are installed, based on the brand being used—generically called multiunit abutments—and then sutured.

This makes it possible to move the prosthesis to a supragingival location, away from the surgical area.

A rubber dam is used to isolate the area and an impression of the temporary prosthesis is taken using addition silicone. This serves a double purpose: copying the position of the abutments and assessing occlusion. The silicone and the acrylic carrying the components are later drilled into, the titanium chimneys are placed on the multiunits and the temporary prosthesis is placed on the area to ensure it fits with the chimneys and the acrylic. After this, it is removed. In the laboratory, it is finished off with acrylic, polished and later installed.

Clinical case

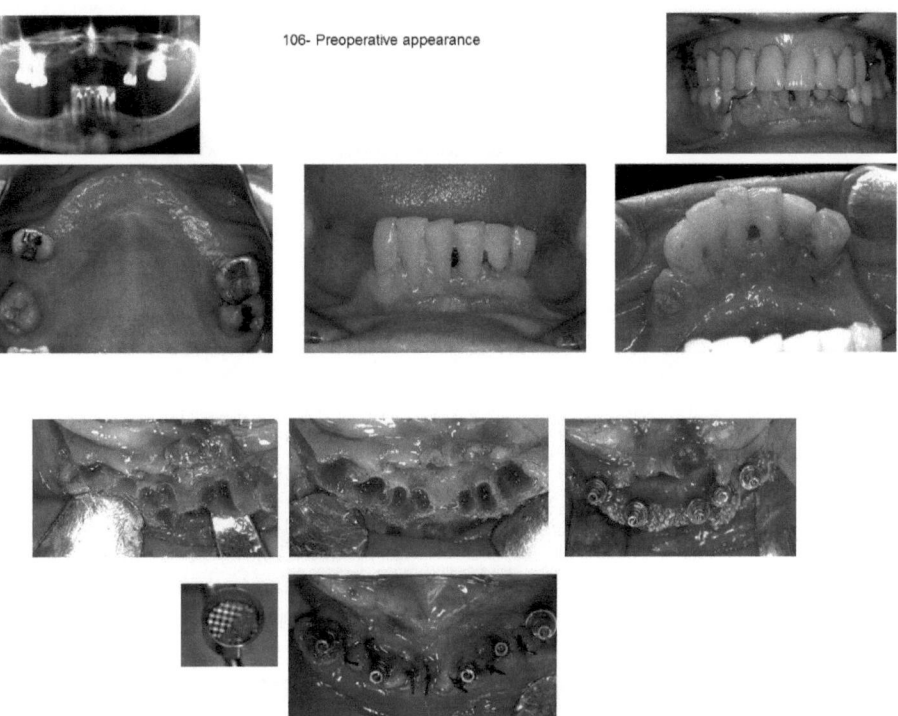

106- Preoperative appearance

107- Surgery. Dental extractions, flattened mandibular bone. Five Biohorizons implants placement and five multiunit

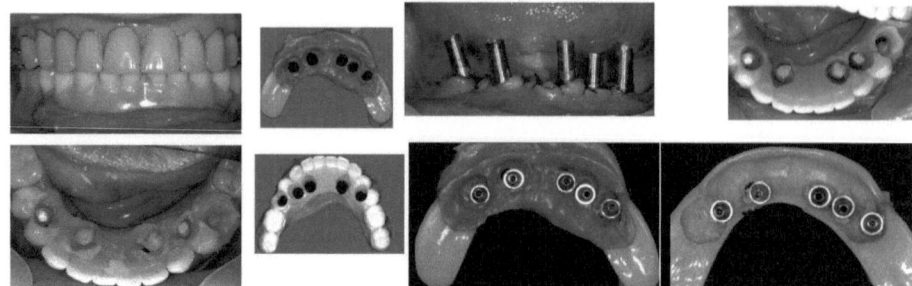

108- Multiunit printing, check occlusal positioning cylinders titanium acrylic fixing the temporary prosthesis

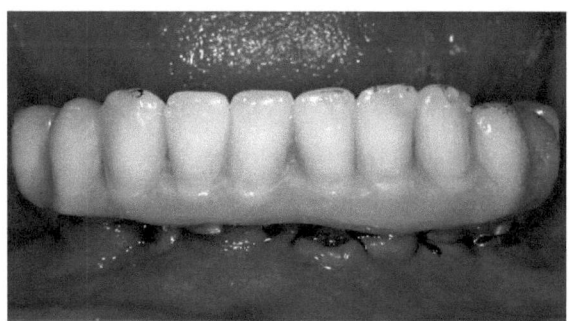

109- Temporary restoration. Hybrid prostheses low complexity

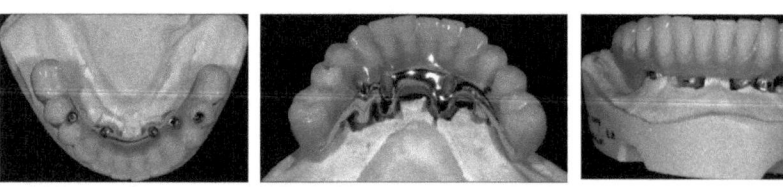

110- Final restoration, hybrid prostheses, medium complexity

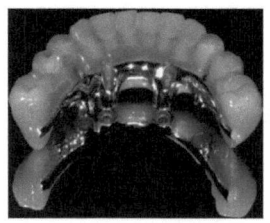
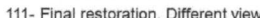
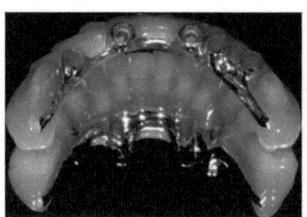
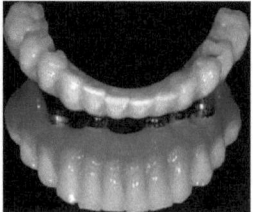

111- Final restoration. Different view

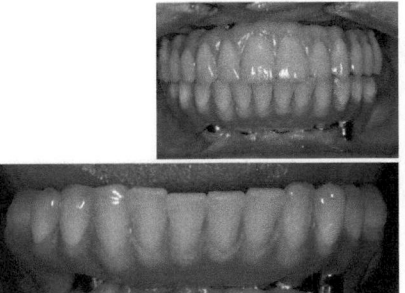
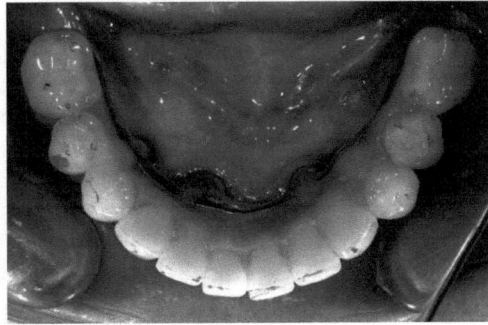

112- Final restoration. Oclussion, vestibular view and occlusal view

Stereolithographics models

In order to understand this technique and for educational purposes, it is first important to appreciate the value of CTs as a diagnostic tool. Together with stereolithographics, it has made it possible to further implantology. Next, we will offer a brief theoretical introduction of the subject, followed by a stage-by-stage case report.

The application of computed tomography (CT) and the use of software for dental implant treatment have increased significantly in recent years. Based on these technologies, implant placement can be guided "partially" or "totally" by the use of splints generated by computer programs and stereolithography that can guide from the osteotomy sequence to implant placement in a three-dimensionally accurate.

The emergence and growing popularity of CT systems with conical collimation (cone beam) allows us to take advantage more and more easily of the different benefits offered by this technology. Among these, obtaining stereolithographic models has become in a very simple and common use procedure that allows us to plan the installation of dental implants and prosthetic design of provisional and definitive restorations.

The aim of this case report is to expand the possibilities offered by CT and stereolithographic models and from which we can obtain accurate information prior to surgical instrumentation and installation of implants and develop prosthetic designs with predictable results.

Introduction

One of the most significant changes in oral implantology has been the growing popularity of immediate loading protocols as a therapeutic alternative in certain circumstances and clinical conditions.

The immediate loading prosthesis has the aim of solving a problem divided into three items: aesthetic, functional and social development from the beginning of its implementation as therapy. To do this, we must establish protocols that simplify and standardize surgical prosthesis for more effective and lasting results.

Traditional planning on clinical, radiographic and laboratory cases, as the study of models and surgical guides are very important to achieve optimal results in the development of our protocols.

The emergence and growing popularity of computed tomography (CT) systems with conical collimation, has improved the diagnosis of dentistry as a whole.

Thanks to these technologies, implantology companies are incorporating implant dentistry guided by CT, which allows installation of prosthetic implants in positions determined preoperatively in the three planes of space as well as provide the ability to place immediate loaded prosthesis.

This paradigm shift from a traditional approach to implant placement to a "computer assisted" includes manufacture of multiple removable guides for drilling to be used exclusively for the preparation of the osteotomy site (ie partially guided) up to use a single fixed guide for osteotomy preparation and installation of the implant (ie fully guided). This technique controls the three planes: buccolingual, mesiodistal and apicocoronal, unlike the partially guided technique that controls the buccolingual and mesiodistal planes, being apicocoronal a surgical calculation.

Another point in the use of CT is obtaining stereolithographic models that reproduce hard tissues with a high degree of accuracy.

The handling of the models in a preoperative stage brings us high value topographic ideas as well as allows perfect surgical simulation through which we can improve the accuracy of traditional surgical guide, achieving a precision technique of conventional intermediate between the guides elaborate on laboratory models and computer assisted.

Clinical case

A 57 –year-old patient with fixed partial denture in jaw from teeth 4.3 to 3.2 combined with removable partial dentures in posterior sector.

Maxilla with natural dentition, absence of 1.6 and 2.4, extrusion of the left posterior with evident signs of tooth wear.

Clinical studies, laboratory studies and radiographic examination were carried out as well as the analysis of articulator mounted models. Standard inclusion criteria were considered for immediate loading protocol in mandibular full arch and computerized tomographic study requested by conical collimating (cone beam) and realization of stereolithographic model of mandible.

Lower plaster model is corrected with removal of teeth and three millimeters of remaining alveolar process (surgery model) to optimize prosthetic space and the lower full dentures are made to be used for the immediate charging procedure.-

The same procedure is performed in the remodeling stereolithographic model, using the same parameters of tooth wear to achieve fixing complete prosthesis on the same range corresponding to the thickness of the mucosa. It is remarkable the stability and adaptation obtained considering that the prosthesis is designed for tissue support and then moved to a surface of bone support.

Two duplicates of the lower denture acrylic translucent are made, then they are checked to have the same settlement than the prosthesis and then they are cut at the lingual sidewall height for the six anterior teeth and the occlusal surface of the four premolars to place in this area five implants to be installed in the interforaminal zone. One of the duplicate will lead the osteotomy guide and the other only large perforations for controlling osteotomies.

Corresponding holes are made in the stereolithographic model and five replicas are installed emerging conical implants with MIS. They are prosthetically guided searching an optimal distribution, maximum distal extent of the support area and ideal emergency to hide the fixing screws. (One implant at middle line, two at each end angled distally and two between the ends and the middle line).

Five cylinders are screwed for immediate loading to the analogs and then they are fixed firmly to a doubling of the prosthesis, with self-curing acrylic. The entire structure is unscrewed, the inside of the cylinders is rectified to eliminate microscrews seat and allow the passage of the initial drill and 2 mm drill during surgical handling. Excesses are cut and polished.

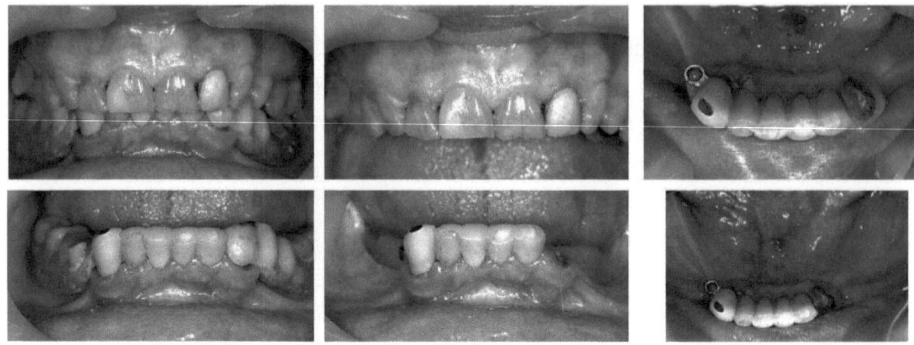

113- Preoperative appearance

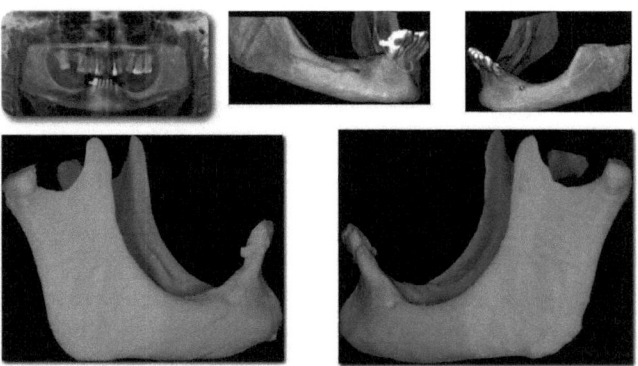

114- Panoramic Rx, cone beam. (mandibular reconstruction). Stereolitographic model complete

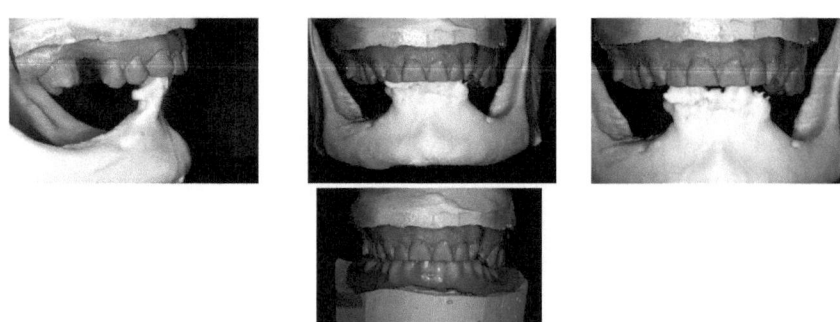

115- Denture provisional design

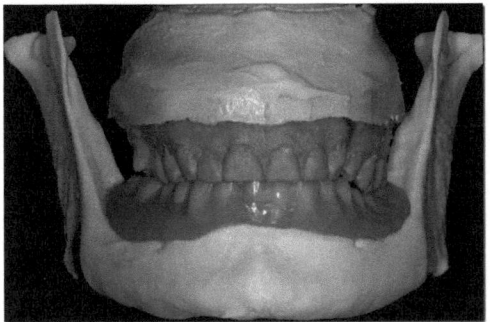

116- Complete denture probe in stereolitographic model

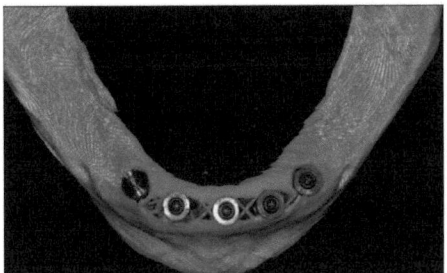

117- Placement multiunit analogin sterolitographic model

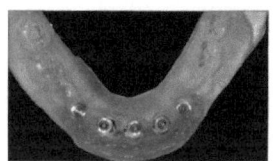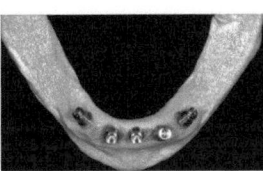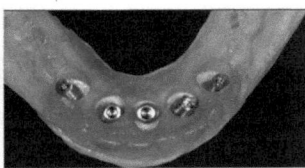

118- Surgical guide preparation (replica of temporary prostheses)

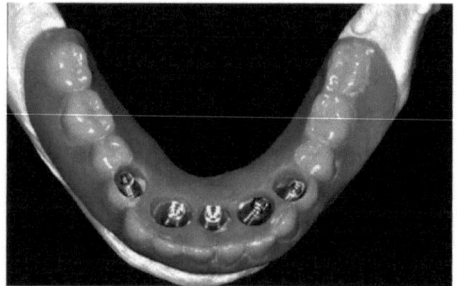

119- Preparation of the temporary prosthesis

Surgical procedures

The extraction of remaining teeth and remodeling of three millimeters of alveolar bone surgery under model are performed. The complete seating of the prosthesis and the maintenance of the planned occlusion are also checked.

Surgical guides are positioned alternately and the osteotomy handlings are performed up to the two millimeters drill. These guides will provide a guidance at mesiodistal and buccolingually. The vertical depth is a surgical calculation and it is not controlled by the guide.

Five MIS implants are installed.

The initial primary stability was evaluated using the torque insertion of the surgical unit and it was recorded according to the recommended classification by Dr Testori et al:

a- TIGHT when torque was> 32 N cm.

b- FIRM between 25 and 32 N cm.

c- LOW N below 25 cm.

Tapered emerging are screwed and soft tissue are stitched.

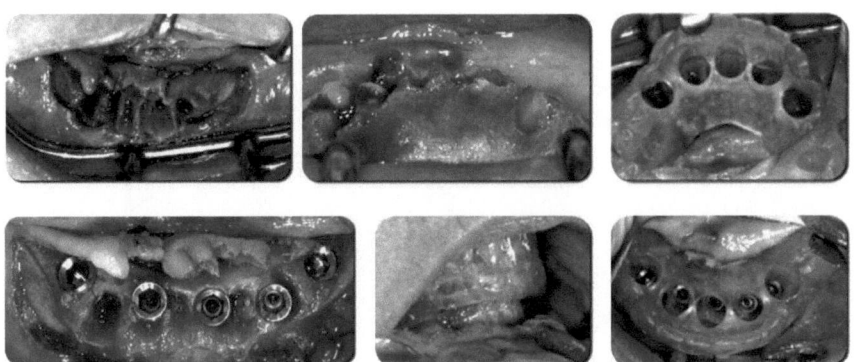

120- Surgery. Five M.I.S implants (seven) trough the surgical guide

Prosthetic procedures

A temporary hybrid prosthesis totally screwed was performed from the following protocol:

The complete prosthesis in the area corresponding to the implants is wore out for the conical emerging not to interfere with proper seating of the same.

Silicone adhesive is placed and is impressed with fluid silicone on the surgical area for the emergency recording of conical component. In addition, silicon improves the stability of the prosthesis during the handling of adhesion of the cylinders as well as insulate soft tissues to avoid acrylic cytotoxicity. Subsequently, areas corresponding to the emerging holes having a sufficient diameter to allow passage of the cylinder in solidarity with the hybrid prosthesis are drilled.

Cylinders are screwed to the conical emerging and the prosthesis is repositioned.

They adhere to the prosthesis cylinders using self-curing acrylic.

Remove the entire assembly, trim and polish the excesses.

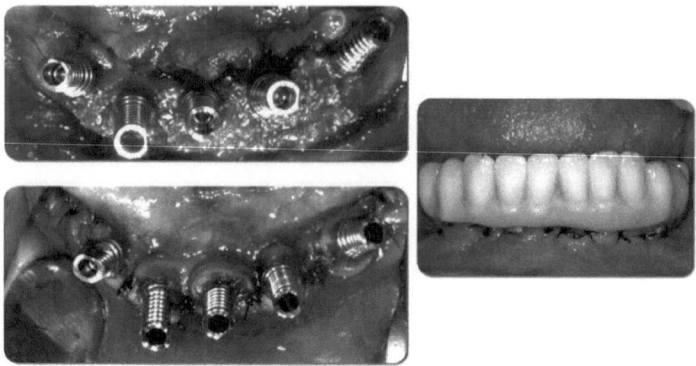

121- Placement Multiunit, temporary cylinders and provisional restoration (Hybrid prostheses low complexity)

Finally the prosthesis is installed, adjusting microscrews in 20 Ncm.

The final prosthetic restoration consists of a highly complex hybrid prosthesis metal ceramics, biomimetic, cemented on machined emerging that are performed at 3 months of immediate loading, after the period of monitoring and verification of osseointegration of implants.

It is clear that stereolithography improves the three-dimensional distribution of implants, therefore planning this way decreases clinical working time, optimizes performance and minimizes surgical trauma, with atraumatic postoperative. Anyway, it is a technique that should still be improved, only the application in different clinical cases and technical modifications, will allow us to evolve and standardize the protocol.

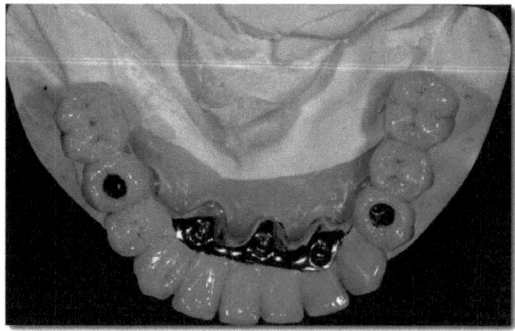

122- Three months later. Preparation of a fixed prosthesis screwed porcelain

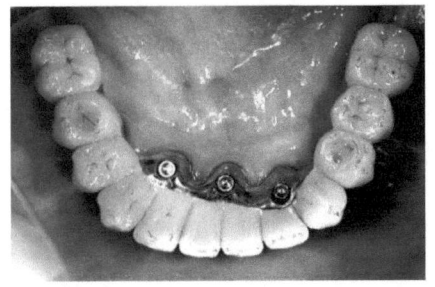 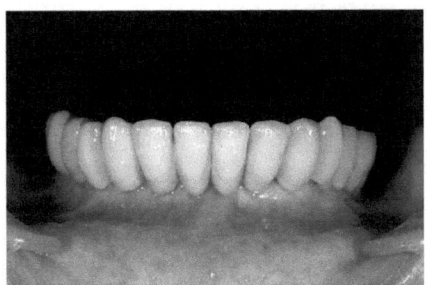

123- Clinical aspects. Occlusal and vestibular view

Conclusion

According to the 2002 Brussels Meeting of the European Osseointegration Academy, using the immediate load technique prevents hard tissue resorption while preserving its architecture.

It is furthermore a highly predictable technique decreasing both post-op trauma and the number of clinical stages necessary.

From a biological standpoint, it also decreases peri-implant, soft tissue loss, particularly when the latter is extremely thin and scalloped, because it undergoes a gradual adaptation process during the integration period: peri-implant tissue is known to experience greater resorption during the first three months (Tarnow 2000-2002), which optimizes aesthetics.

Lastly, it can be said that the creation of protocols and their standardization minimizes the number of surgical steps necessary, and yields better and more lasting results. Moreover, once they have become standardized, protocols tend to recur and stabilize, which means they can be used by a wide range of professionals, thus increasing their significance as a technique.

BIBLIOGRAPHY

1) Albrektsson, T., Zarb, G., Worthington, P. & Ericksson, A.R. (1986) The Long – Term Efficacy of Currrently Used Dental Implants: A Review and Proposed Criteria for Success, International Journal of Oral Maxillofacial Implants I: 11-25.

2) Babbush, C. A., Kent, J. & Misiek, D, (1986). Titanium Plasma – Sprayed (TPS) Screw Implants for the Reconstruction of the Edentulous Mandible. Journal of oral Maxillofacial Surgery 44: 274-282.

3) Baker, D. A., London, R.M. & O'Neil, R. B. (1999) Rate of Pull–Out Strength Gain of Dual Etched Titanium Implants: A Comparative Study in Rabbits, International Journal of Oral Maxillofacial Implants I 4: 722-728.

4) Balshi, T.J. & Wolfinger, G.J. (1997) Immediate Loading of Branemark Implants in Edentulous Mandibles: A Preliminary Report. Implant Dentistry 6: 63-88.

5) Branemark, P. I., Hansson , B. O., Adell, R., Breine, U., Lindström, J., Hallen, O. & Öhamn, A. (I997) Osseointegrated Implants in the Treatment of the Edentulous Jaw. Experience from a 10-Year Period. Scandinavian Journal of Plastic and Reconstructive Surgery I6: I-I32.

6) Buser, D., Mericske- Stem, R., Bernard, J.P, Behnecke, A., Belnecke, N., Hirt, H.P., Belser, U.C. & N.P. (I997). Long–Term Evaluation of Nonsubmerged Titanium Implants. I. 8–Year Life Table Analysis of a Prospective Multi–Center Study with 2359 Implants. Clinical Oral Implants Research 8: I6I –172.

7) Chaushu, G., S., Tzohar, A.& Dayan , D. (200I). Immediate Loading of Single– Tooth Implants: Immediate Versus Non–Immediate Implantation. A Clinical Report. International Journal of Oral Maxillofacial Implants I6: 267 –272.

8) Chiapasco, M, Gatti, C., Rossi, E., Haefliger, W. & Markwalder, T. H. (I997) Implants Retained Mandibular Overdentures with Immediate Loading. A Retrospective Multicenter Study on 226 Consecutive Cases. Clinical Oral Implants Research 8: 48-57.

9) Cochran, D.L., Schenk, R.K., Lussi, A., Higginbottom, & Buser , D. (I998) Bone Response to Unloaded and Loaded Titanium Implants with a Sandblasted and

Acid Etched Surface : A Histometric Study in the Canine Mandible. Journal of Biomedical Material Research 40: 1-11.

10)   Cordioli, G., Majzoub , Z., Piattelli, A. & Scarano, A. (2000) Removal Torque and Histomorphometric Investigation of 4 Different Titanium Surfaces: An Experimental Study in the Rabbit Tibia. International Journal of Oral Maxillofacial Implants I6: 668-674.

11)   Darvanapah, M., Martínez, H. & Tecucianu, J. F. (2000), Apical–Coronal Position: Recent Surgical Proposals. Technical Note. International Journal of Oral Maxillofacial Implants I5: 865-872.

12)   Ericson, I., Nilson , H., Lindhe, J., Nilner, K, K. & Randow, K. (2000ª= Immediate Functional Loading of Branemark Single Tooth Implants. An 18 months´ Follow–Up Study. Clinical Oral Implants Research II: 26-33.

13)   Ericson, I, Randow, K., Nilner , K. & Peterson, A. (2000b) Early Functional Loading of Branemark Dental Implants. 5 Year Clinical Follow–Up Study. Clinical Implant Dentistry Related Research 2: 70-77.

14)   Klokkeold n, P.R., Nishimura n, R. D., Adachi , M & Caputo , A. M. (I997) Osseointegration Enhanced by Chemical Etching of the Titanium Surface. A Torque Removal Study in the Rabbit. Clinical Oral Implants Research 8: 442-447.

15)   Lermann, P. D., (I979) Stegprothestische Versorgung des Zahnlosen Unterkiefers mit Hilfe plasmabeschichtete Unterkiefers mit Hilfe plasmabeschichteten Titanschraubimplantaten. Deutsche Zahnärtzliche Zeitung 34: 907-9II.

16)   Leklolm, U. & Zarb, G. A. (I985) Patient Selection and Preparation. In Branemark, P. –I., Zarb, G.A. & Albrektsson, T., eds. Tissue Integrated Prosthesis: Osseointegration in Clinical Dentistry, 199- 209. Chicago: Quintessence Publishing Co.

17)   Lozada, J. L., Tsukamoto, N, Farnos, A., Kan, J, & Rungcharassaeng , K. (2000) Scientific Rationale for the Surgical and Prosthodontic Protocol for Immediately Loaded Root Form Implants in the Completely Edentulous Patient. Journal of Oral Implantology 26: 5I-58.

18) Schnitman, P., Wöhrle, P. S., & Rubenstein, J.E. (I990) Immediate Fixed Interim Prostheses Supported by Two–Stage Threaded Implants: Methodology and Results. Journal of Oral Implantology 2: 96-105.

19) Schnitman, P., Wöhrle, P.S., Rubenstein, J.E., DaSilva, J.D. & Wang, N.H. (I997) Ten Years´ Results for Branemark Implants Immediately Loaded with Fixed Prostheses Implant Placement. International Journal of Oral Maxillofacial Implants I6: 495-503.

20) Schroeder, A., Maeglin, B. & Sutter, F. (I993) Das ITI- Hohlzy Limderimplantat Typ F zur Prosthesen-retention beim zahnlosen Kiefer. Schweizersche Monastschrift fur Zahnheikunde 93: 720-733.

21) Szmukler – Moncler, S., (2000) Considerations Preliminary to the Application of Early and Immediate Loading Protocols in Dental Implantology, Clinical Oral Implants Research II: 12 – 25.

22) Tarnow, D. P., Emtiaz, S. & Classi, A., (I997) Immediate Loading of Threaded Implants at Stage I Surgery in Edentulous Arches: Ten Consecutive Case Reports with 1- to 5- Year Data. International Journal of Oral Maxillofacial Implants I2: 3I9-324.

23) Tesori, T., Francetti, L., Del Fabro, M., Zuffetti, C. & Weinstein, R. L.(I999) A Radiographic Evaluation of Crestal bone Changes in Submerged Implants Supra and Sub–Crestally Positioned. A Pilot Study in Humans. Clinical Oral Implants Research I0: 178 (Abstract).

24) Testori, T, Szmukler – Moncler, Sm, Francetti, L., Del Fabbro, M., Scarano A., Piattelli, A & Weinstein, R. L. (200Ia) Immediate Loading of Osseotite Implants. A Case Report and Histologic Analysis after 4 Months of Occlusal Loading. International Journal of Periodontics Restorative Dentistry 2I: 451-459.

25) Testori, T., Szmukler – Moncler, S., Francetti, L., Del Fabbro, M., Trisi, P. & Weinstein, R. L. (2002b) Healing of Osseotite Implants under Submerged and Immediate Loading Conditions in a Patient: A Case Report and Interface Analysis

after 2 Months. International Journal of Periodontics Restorative Dentistry 22: 345-353.

26) Testori, T., Wiseman, L., Woolfe, S. & Porter, S.S. (200Ib) A Prospective Multicenter Clinical Study of the Osseotite Implant: Four–Year Interim Report. International Journal of Oral Maxillofacial Implants I6: 193 – 200.

27) Trisi, P. & Rao, W. (I999) Bone Classification: Clinical–Histomorphometric Comparison. Clinical Oral Implants Research I0: 1-7.

28) Trisi, P., Rao, W. & Rebaudi, A. (I999) A Histometric Comparison of Smooth and Rough Titanium Implants in Human Low Density Jaw-Bone. International Journal of Oral Maxillofacial Implants I4: 698-698.

29) Reducción de los Tiempos Clínicos en Prótesis Implantoasistida. Revista de la Asociación Odontológica Argentina. Vol. 88 N.° 1, pp. 35-40. enero/febrero de 2000.

30) Carga inmediata en arcos completos Maxilar inferior. Libro Carga inmediata en Prótesis implantoasistida. Bases Bilógicas. Aplicaciones terapéuticas (2008). Capítulo 2: 32-53.

31) Testori, T, Meltler A, Troiano Miguel, et Al (2004) Inmediate Occlusal Loading of Osseotite Implants in the Lower Edentolous Jaw. A Multicenter Prospective Study Clinical Oral Implant Research 15; 278- 284.

32) Albertini G, Cagnone G, Troiano M. Simplified protocol using a translucent transference guide (T.T.G.) in immediate implant loading in the edentolous mandible. Annals of Oral & Maxillofacial Surgery 2013 Dec 21;1(4):36.

33) Troiano M. Prospective multicentre study of immediate occlusal loading of implants in edentulous mandibles. Annals of Oral & Maxillofacial Surgery 2013 Feb 01;1(1):6.

34) Troiano M, Sanchez P, Benincasa M, Cagnone G. Correct use of artificial gum for implant-assisted prosthesis. Annals of Oral & Maxillofacial Surgery 2013 Jun 01;1(2):19.

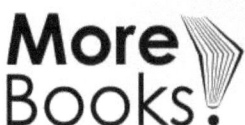
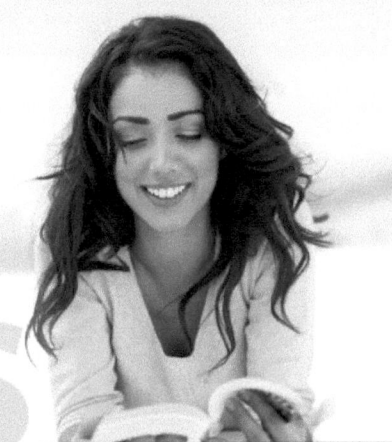

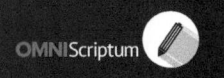

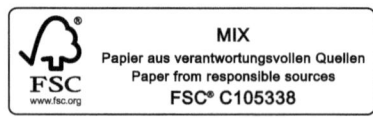
Printed by Books on Demand GmbH, Norderstedt / Germany